One Woman's Journey Through Chronic Pain,
Depression, Addiction and Back Again

Athlete on Oxy

D0869090

Erin Johnson

outskirts
press

For Todd, Lexi, Mom and Dad

Table of Contents

Author's Note

Addiction versus Dependency

I really struggle with calling myself an addict. Was I addicted to OxyContin? Physically, yes. Psychologically, no. Did I enjoy the effects of the drug on my brain, pain relief notwithstanding? Yes. But I knew I couldn't take them forever. During my time on opioids I behaved like an addict, counting pills and thinking about drugs all the time. Making sure I knew where those white tablets of bliss were and when I needed to take them to maintain pain relief. I was also hyper-aware of how much I needed to take to avoid the symptoms of acute withdrawal which started about ten hours after taking a dose. That sure sounds like addiction. But here is where I struggle—I've taken opioids since beating my addiction to Oxy, once for a toothache and again for a bike accident. And when I took them it was no big deal—I didn't want to drop everything and binge on pills. I took them until they were gone. That was it, end of story. This fact separates me from many others who have experienced addiction. So, I often call myself opioid dependent in this book out of respect for those who can never touch their drug(s) again for fear they could, at best, fall back into bad patterns, and at worst, kill themselves. I'm not trying to portray myself as better than any other addict, I just want to respect the word and all that it means. I am not living under the illusion that I was anything less than addicted to Oxy.

The Characters

I asked a handful of people to share their perspectives on certain aspects of my story. You will see their words interwoven throughout this book. The purpose of adding their thoughts was not to substantiate my views or offer support of my character. It was really to get raw, honest feedback about their experiences as they relate to me.

In order of appearance:

Jen – my therapist
Dr. Omer – hip preservation surgeon
Mom – egg provider
Keira – oldest Boulder friend
Jen – best friend since college
Heidi – best friend in Boulder
Dad – sperm provider
Dr. MK – diagnostic specialist
Todd – my husband
Rico – owner, Streetside Dance Studio

Financial Privilege

I was fortunate enough to have access to highly respected doctors throughout my decade of pain and surgery. I had health insurance. I lived in an upper middle-class neighborhood surrounded by my small, loving and supportive family. I realize that I was lucky—my journey may have looked very different if I had not had access to top-notch healthcare. If it was this hard for me to find answers to my pain mystery and beat addiction, what would it look like for someone who could not just quit their job because they wanted to, or for a single parent or someone without health insurance? I'm telling this story as it unfolded for me. I don't believe that everyone shares these resources, but I do believe that it is our job as a nation to work towards equitable healthcare for everyone.

Foreword

When I started this project, I wasn't exactly sure what I wanted to accomplish. And even over halfway through my first rough draft I still wasn't sure. Was this a memoir, or just an act of catharsis? Was it about chronic pain, or our broken healthcare system? Was it about opioids, or grit and determination? Was it about surviving and fighting, or the importance of friends and family? The truth is it's about all of those things. I couldn't just pick one purpose or one overarching theme that I thought would resonate with every human. It's my hope that you will read something in these pages that resonates with you. I hope you will read something that will make you more vulnerable to the human condition, because truth be told, I'm not the only one to ever fall on hard times. There are certainly many people out there with way bigger health problems than I will ever have and there are many people out there who will never have a similar experience. But you know what, we all have our own struggles. You are on your own path.

Often when friends or acquaintances are telling me their stories, they'll stop and say something like "I know you've been through so much more...so I probably sound kind of stupid...my problems aren't nearly as bad as yours were." And I always respond the same way— we only know what we know. We only know our own experiences, and if it's hard for you, then it's hard for you. You don't have to quantify your pain, whether it's physical or emotional, for me or for anyone else. You get to be you and your journey is yours to experience.

So, while you're reading or listening to my story, just know I don't think I'm any worthier of writing a memoir than anyone else. These pages are full of my life lessons, and I hope that in them you'll find a nugget of wisdom you can use to get through whatever challenges life throws at you, because you better believe those challenges, they are coming.

Control

We make decisions all the time, every day. Each choice we make leads us to the next moment—decision then outcome, decision, outcome, over and over. We make choices every minute of every day and most of them go unnoticed.

I get up in the morning and get dressed, I am warm. I drink coffee, I feel awake. I eat breakfast, I am full. Each action has a somewhat predictable reaction, an end result that keeps me moving forward. Each choice moves me into the next choice. I can choose each action and most of the time, predict the subsequent effect. That surely feels like control.

Of course, these are just the small choices I make. I also make big choices. I choose to work hard on a project for work and then finish. I do research on a particular topic of interest and I learn. I train hard for a race or event and I complete it. I feel in control of my life. What are some of the choices you made today? Does your day look like you expected? Maybe something didn't go as planned. Maybe your son or daughter was sick. Maybe your car wouldn't start. Maybe you forgot your lunch. But you knew how to adjust to all of those little events, even if it was annoying. It wasn't that hard.

But, what if everything you ever thought about cause and effect, adjusting to change, all just evaporated? And not just in one critical moment, like a car crash or a natural disaster, but over a period of many years. What if, for eight years, you couldn't adjust, life did not make sense, and each decision you thought was the right one, with a predictable effect, did not give you the outcome you anticipated?

For example, what if you got out of bed and got dressed but could never get warm? What if you drank endless amounts of coffee and never felt awake? What if you ate breakfast but never felt full? What if everything you ever thought about your choices and how you could direct your life was just gone? What if every choice you thought was GOOD led to a WORSE place? What happens when you realize that control is an illusion? How would you handle it?

In 2010, I still believed I was in control of my life.

PART ONE
FOREPLAY

CHAPTER 1

NFL AFC Championship Game 2015

MY DAUGHTER, LEXI, and I are at the nail salon. I'm getting my nails painted alternating blue and orange today. My football team, the Denver Broncos, are in the playoffs against the New England Patriots. My husband, Todd, and I would surely be going to see them play at Invesco Field—if I wasn't dopesick.

My insides churn as the smell of nail polish remover roils my stomach. My head feels like it will explode at any minute. And I am just hoping, praying that I don't throw up all over the place, embarrassing my daughter. I don't want to explain to these people that I have been taking opioid pain medication for years and yesterday I stopped. I try hard to pretend everything is okay giving my daughter hugs and smiles as we have this fun bonding experience together. But I am dizzy and sick. I feel my eyes rolling into the back of my head and think I'm going to faint. If I can just get some fresh air, I'll be okay. That's when I jump out of the reclining pedicure chair and push out the door. I stand over the bushes lining the strip mall and dry heave. I assure Lexi there is nothing to see here, I'm just not feeling great.

It has been less than twenty-four hours since I took my last OxyContin.

The day goes on in a blur as I assure my friends and family that I'm fine and withdrawal "isn't that bad." I lie on my couch surrounded by Todd, Lexi and my parents watching the much-anticipated football game, but my mind is not right. I can't focus on the television, on what is happening in front of me because my brain feels like scrambled eggs and I can't get comfortable. My legs seem to move on their own, like they're not attached to my body. I keep staring at my fingernails—orange and blue—but they're out of focus and I'm sick. I can't eat the tailgate-style meal I prepared and I can't even remember cooking anything. I wonder if anyone around me can tell that something is so very wrong with me. Can they see how hard this is? Can they see this mom, daughter and wife coming apart right before their eyes?

I know the Broncos won that game, but I can't remember one play. I just remember how I felt, alone and scared. Scared of what was to come and alone in my fight to break the hold these opioids had on me. I knew I was not going to die, but I wondered if I would ever be the same person on the other side of all this mess. I wondered if something would break inside me and I would find myself ordering pills online or searching for the feeling of blissful indifference in the back alleys of Denver. I was still in pain, but I couldn't assess the reality of it anymore. Two months earlier I had the fourth surgery on my hip. It was a hip replacement and in theory I should be just fine. But I still hurt every single day. It hurt to walk. It hurt to get up. It hurt to stand. It hurt all the time. But not as much as it did before the replacement, I thought.

Right?
It hurt less, right?
Yes. Less.
Wait, no. I think it still hurts the same.
Worse.
No. Yes?
I'm not sure.

This was me every day post replacement—I had no idea what was real anymore. The doctors told me everything looked great. But how could I really know anything about anything taking OxyContin around the clock? I couldn't. I had to get off the drugs and figure out if the pain was real or not. I had to figure out what was real, period. What started as a Vicodin every afternoon had exploded into a full-blown dependency on OxyContin.

Night proved to be the worst—sleep was nowhere to be found. I spent the night in a place of sleep purgatory somewhere between consciousness and unconsciousness, lying in bed sweating and twisting in the sheets. There was no rest to be had, only constant motion and discomfort. My head was pounding, a drum beat of pain against my temples. I didn't know when or if it would ever stop. I moved from the mattress to the bathroom floor several times waiting for the vomit churning in my stomach to erupt, but it never did. It was like having the worst flu imaginable and it was never going to get better. There was no medicine I could take to help me move through this experience. I just had to accept it and be in it, 100% unequivocally in it.

I wondered if there were some pills somewhere in the house, a Percocet or Vicodin, maybe even an Oxy I had dropped between the couch cushions. Or maybe one had slipped out of my handbag and landed on the floor of my car—I carried my pills with me everywhere. But in all honesty, I knew there were none. I had already combed the couch cushions and floor boards of the car for pills before. I had found them all and there were none left. I didn't really want to take any more pain killers at that moment anyway. And that's the truth. But I did want the symptoms of withdrawal to stop. No one had prepared me for this. My pain doctor made it sound like if I tapered, it would be no big deal. But it was a big deal, a huge deal. Lying there on the cold tile covered in a bath towel I wondered, "How did I get here... how on earth is this my life?"

CHAPTER 2

Thirty-Five Years in a Nutshell

TO FULLY GRASP the journey I am about to share with you, you have to understand where I came from, how I grew up and what led me to believe the things I did about life. So, stay with me for a brief history lesson.

As a child and for much of my young adult life, I had everything. I was pretty, smart, athletic, popular, loved and healthy. For most of my life, I really had it all.

Born to solid middle-class parents in 1973, I entered their lives most unexpectedly. My mother had a severe case of endometriosis and was told it was very unlikely she would be able to have children. When she did get pregnant, it was nothing short of a miracle for her and my father. They knew how lucky they were and there was no question that they would do anything necessary to make sure I lived a full and wonderful life. My mom stayed home with me and worked part-time jobs on and off throughout my childhood. My dad was a high school government teacher and a gifted coach.

I was a loving kid with a fierce drive to compete. I had been a top-level rhythmic gymnast for much of my young life, laying the foundation for my future athletic endeavors. You may be thinking, "What the hell is rhythmic gymnastics?" When people ask me, I always say, "Have you ever seen the sport in the Olympics where the girl dances with a ribbon?" Yep, that's it.

I thrived on competition and was willing to put in serious work. I understood what it meant to win—and not by chance, by earning it. I carried this lesson into the rest of my life. In high school I was a straight-A student, member of the National Honor Society, assistant captain of the pom-pom squad and photography editor of the yearbook. When I graduated my fellow classmates had nominated me "Most Likely to Be Miss Clairol," "Best Dressed" and "Best Physique."

My parents said that if I graduated with a GPA above 3.5, I could go to any college I wanted. They totally should have known better... with a kid like me, there was no way I would not achieve this goal.

So instead of going to a Missouri school to party, take drugs, follow the Grateful Dead and Phish and generally waste my education, I went two states over and my parents paid 50% more for me to do just that. Now that I am an adult, I really can't believe how much I took all that for granted. And on top of it, I stayed for FIVE years and got a degree in...wait for it...Parks and Recreation.

The one good thing about my college experience is I discovered my love for the outdoors there. I took an Adventure Recreation class as an elective when I was a Poly Sci/Philosophy major. For spring break we went out to Utah for some rock climbing, backpacking, camping and general outdoor fun. Upon arrival in Moab, Utah I was immediately smitten. I had never been west of Missouri and had no idea what the rest of the United States was like. I couldn't believe the natural beauty of the landscape and the peace it made me feel inside. Sleeping under the stars became the favorite place to lay my head. And being active in the outdoors became my church. I felt closest to God in nature, so much more so than I ever had in a church growing up. I had found my place of worship and it was all around me.

When I returned from that trip, I promptly changed my major to Parks and Rec and envisioned a life like Edward Abby, roaming the desert writing prose and smoking weed. In 1996 my parents and grandparents supported me doing a National Outdoor Leadership School semester in the Southwest. During this experience the group backpacked for forty days, rock climbed for fifteen days, canoed down the Rio Grande for seventeen days and explored underground caverns for thirteen days. In total we slept outside for ninety days and took four showers. It was so awesome! I loved the simplicity of my life, getting from point A to point B, never looking in a mirror and relying on myself for everything. I learned so much about the desert Southwest and saw the natural world in a most pristine way. It was heaven!

Unfortunately, because I had always been granted every opportunity from my parents, I had no idea what real life after college would be like. And man, that was a rude awakening. I had two jobs out of college—working at an outdoor gear store called JL Waters and leading rock climbing trips for the Indiana University Outfitters. Neither paid well, but I didn't care that much. I was happy. And I knew from the moment I saw the Rocky Mountains for the first time that I wanted to live there someday. But being a relatively sheltered girl from the Midwest, I wasn't sure exactly how I would ever get there.

And then the one thing that can make you do just about anything came waltzing into my life. LOVE.

Steve was my first "adult" love. We spent two years together in college. One week before college graduation Steve broke my heart. He had fallen out of love with me and was ready for a change. Shortly after, he packed his bags and moved to…yep, sunny Boulder, Colorado. So, when he came crawling back a year later to say breaking up with me was the biggest mistake he had ever made, I melted. Within six months I had packed my Ford Explorer and headed for the promised land.

I got a job at the Boulder Mountaineer in the heart of the college part of town. Everyone who worked there was bad-ass. Climbing legends such as Lynn Hill and Bobbi Bensmen had worked there and I was following in their footsteps. I talked about rock climbing, trail running, tele skiing and backpacking all day. It was great—I felt like I had found my place in the world.

Eventually I was promoted to Apparel Buyer. I LOVED this job.

It was so much fun. I got to review all of the products made by Patagonia, The North Face, Marmot, Mountain Hardwear, Prana, etc. and then decide which styles were best for our store. It was fabulous and I was very good at it. But, after a few years thriving in the Apparel Buyer job, I began to feel stuck, like I wasn't going anywhere with my life. I was broke and bored. So, I decided to pursue something I knew I would be good at—graduate school.

I applied and was accepted (thank God for the GMAT scores and letters of recommendations to offset a degree in Parks and Rec), to the School of Business at the University of Colorado at Denver. During the time I pursued my MBA, I took several classes in Entrepreneurship. In one of those classes we were challenged to develop a new business opportunity. I pored over ideas on how to make the poorly paying job I adored something I could actually do as a "real job." In the process of doing this I came up with an idea that would serve as the REAL beginning of my twenty-year career buying outdoor clothing for living.

From one of these entrepreneurship classes, Outdoor Apparel Insights was born. Since I had become a very proficient apparel buyer over the years, it was taking me less and less time to do my job. It wasn't really a full-time gig anymore. So I thought, what if I was able to bring economies of scale to the local mom and pop outdoor shop? What if I could provide them with a professional buying service for less than it would cost to hire a full-time buyer? Brilliant, right? I got my first client outside of Boulder in 2000, a store called Mountain Miser located in Englewood, Colorado. The owner, David, was young and hot. We hit it off right away!

Other clients followed—some good, some bad—but I always had work doing something I loved. Like any job, it wasn't perfect, but the positive far outweighed the negative. I traveled all over Colorado visiting and staying in some of the most beautiful places on earth including Aspen, Vail and Buena Vista. But the very best thing about this job was the flexibility to work from home and create my own schedule. I could play in the Colorado mountains just about whenever I wanted.

When I wasn't doing this fabulous job I was climbing, Nordic skiing, trail running and mountain biking. I spent most of my time in Boulder being a sort of "jack of all trades." So, when I randomly happened upon a ridiculous sport called adventure racing, I found I had the perfect skill set. The sport was "in vogue" for a short time in the early to mid 2000's. It was, and still is, a very expensive sport. You have to purchase tons of gear and have tons of time on your hands to do some crazy training, like, for example, riding your bike fifty miles to the base of a Colorado mountain that is 14,000 feet tall, climbing it and then riding home...oh yeah, and all in the dark. SO MUCH FUN!

Adventure races are generally multi-sport endeavors where groups of four spend several days navigating through the mountains and rivers of a given area. The teams generally don't sleep much or rest because the first team to complete the multi-day course wins. I had a great team, and I was the only female on it. At the time I was very strong on my feet and in the boat, but a weak mountain bike rider. Our team trained relentlessly and had an amazing time pushing our bodies to the absolute limit. At one point we even had Whole Foods as a sponsor for one of our bigger races—very cool.

After my adventure racing days were over I turned my athletic focus to ultra-distance mountain biking. I entered my first 100-mile mountain bike race in 2002, the Leadville 100. I spent a lot of time on my bike training for this race and became quite a proficient rider. My ability to suffer on the bike was fantastic. And I loved it—the pain, the sweat, the journey to achieving a goal. Back then, I often thought, I was born to do this. My legs would feel so powerful, my cadence smooth and the scenery was always amazing. Training and racing in Colorado is awesome. Everyone is so good, it pushed me to be better. And better I got.

I finished sixth overall at the Leadville 100 that year, and was totally hooked on this sport. Over the next five years I would take first place in the Laramie Enduro, second overall at the now defunct Vail 100, and fourth and fifth respectively at the Breckenridge 100.

In 2006 I received a professional mountain biking license from USA cycling and started a year of racing with the big guns. I was so grateful for my flexible schedule, my cool job and the absolutely unbelievable, fantastic life I had created. It was all so good, even I want to barf right now writing about it.

The only thing missing was a man to share it with.

Don't get me wrong, my life was full of males. To quote a psychic I saw once in New Orleans, "I see many, many men in your life." And she was right. I worked in an industry dominated by men, competed with men and dated men—lots of them.

Generally speaking I was attracted to a bit of a bad boy. I think many people go through a bad boy phase. I kind of took that phase and really dragged it out well into my late twenties. And by then they aren't really bad boys any more, but rather men with no real job, no future, no house and generally no purpose other than to have fun, explore and adventure. I loved that, the thrill of it all. But it didn't pay the bills or provide the stability I craved for my future. Then I met Todd Johnson.

He worked for one of my clients, Ute Mountaineer, in Aspen, Colorado. I met him my first day on the job three years before we started dating. I thought he was adorable and funny. As time went on we developed a friendship and I saw him monthly during my visits to the store. He enjoyed listening to my man drama and I enjoyed flirting with him. Then one weekend he and a couple of his friends came to Boulder for a bike race and they stayed at my condo. One thing led to another and we ended up making out for most of the night (needless to say he dropped out of that bike race the next day). I thought it was fun, but when the boys headed back to Aspen, I thought nothing of it.

But he called. Every. Single. Day. And at first, I was like, why are you calling me? And he would say, "just to talk," and then he would talk and talk and talk. He would ask questions and we would tell stories. It was fun and after a while I thought, wow, I think I really like this guy. And that was the beginning of the most amazing relationship of my life.

Todd and I had a wonderful time together and dated long distance for nine months before he proposed, at about midnight on December 13, 2004. And I said yes.

Our wedding was picture perfect. We got married outside on a beautiful fall day in Crested Butte, Colorado. Sixty of our closest friends and family attended what I thought was the most amazing ceremony. The entire thing was not planned or rehearsed. We had no idea what our officiants were going to say or what our vows would be. Everything was a surprise and it was the most beautiful thirty minutes of my life. Love poured out of everyone there, tears flowed, and I knew that this was perfect, absolutely perfect.

Our wedding was in the morning and followed by brunch. After eating, Todd and I and twenty of our closest friends set out on a four-hour mountain bike ride. Not everyone made it the whole way, but those who did shared an awesome experience with us. That night we had a pizza party at the Secret Stash, an iconic Crested Butte restaurant full of wacky art and Buddha statues. We sat on giant cushions on the floor, drank beer and ate brownies. It was a magical day. Maybe not every girl's dream wedding, but it sure was mine.

Fun and happiness filled the next two years. Todd moved from Aspen into my condo and shortly after we bought our first house in Louisville, Colorado. We spent most of our time working fun outdoor industry jobs and racing our bikes. I had become a great technical rider and a contender in most ultra-distance mountain bike races. I loved training—I loved getting faster and stronger. I loved the days when I felt unstoppable. I once ran into former road cycling legend, Tyler Hamilton, in the Boulder foothills in March. It was freezing, snowing and my toes were numb. I had stopped in Ward, a small mountain town that has a general store with great homemade chocolate chip cookies. It was just Tyler and me up there and I thought, "how bad ass am I right now?" It was a great feeling. I was so tough. I had this great job that allowed me the flexibility to train, a gorgeous husband and a new home in *Money* magazine's best small town in America. What more could I ask for?

CHAPTER 3

Lexi

HOW ABOUT STARTING a family? I was now thirty-three years old and not getting any younger. Todd and I both wanted at least two kids, so we figured it was time to start trying. So, I went off birth control and voilà—in two months I was pregnant.

I hated being pregnant. It sucked. I remember right when I found out, I thought I would go for a short three-mile trail run to celebrate. It was an easy run I would have done with no problem before conception. But it was like an alien had hijacked my body—I couldn't breathe, and could barely run at all. I was so tired. Every limb felt weak. I walked, and this did not make me happy. I didn't have any friends who had children, so I had no idea what pregnancy would be like. I didn't think I would be so tired all the time. I was exhausted and pretty much gave up exercise for the first three months. I couldn't ride my bike, it made me so nauseous. And then there was the food thing…

I had virtually no body fat before I got pregnant, so the first thing I did was gain about twenty pounds in the first three months. Even my obstetrician was like "Erin, you really need to watch what you eat during pregnancy. At this rate, you'll gain well over the recommended twenty-five to thirty-five pounds." Translation: I was going to be very fat, very soon. But I could not stop myself from eating. My favorite snack—yes, snack—was an Einstein's sausage, egg and cheese bagel. It called to me at least three or four days a week.

Fortunately, once I gained that twenty pounds, only five more followed during the rest of the pregnancy, leaving me at the low end of the recommended weight gain. Needless to say, I was very happy with this. I stayed active after those initial three months running, climbing, hiking and lifting weights until well into my 35th week. I thought to myself, I got this, and as soon as this baby is born everything will go back to "normal." I had no plans for child care. I thought, I'll work while the baby sleeps, no big deal. I also thought I would just bring the baby with me on my travels for work. She'll (did I mention it's a girl?) just sleep in the car and hang out in the pack and play at the retail stores where I work. That's what it's for, right?

We had bought literally everything that is supposed to make a baby happy—bouncy seats, swings, a pack and play, toys, stuffed animals and blankets. I remember going to Babies 'R' Us and spending hundreds and hundreds of dollars on all this crap. I bought everything that had four stars on the rating scale. This was going to be one happy, happy baby.

Oh, how wrong I would be.

After forty-two weeks of pregnancy I was so ready for this child to be out of my body. I had a lovely birth plan that included my natural child birth, no drugs, just me and Todd getting through it together. It was going to be beautiful...and it was.

On June 25, 2008 I started having contractions around 10 p.m. I slept fitfully until around 5 a.m. when we decided this was indeed the real deal. We went for a walk around the open space close to our house and fantasized about what our new life would be like with our baby girl. We had decided to name her Alexis (but we would call her Lexi) Claire (after Todd's grandmother) Johnson. We were so excited. After returning home we called the doctor and they told us to come in to see how dilated I was. Turns out I was at seven centimeters upon arrival and ready to be admitted to the hospital. I labored with my husband for seventeen hours total. And up until that point in my life, I had never really known pain. I thought about some of the ultra-distance mountain bike races I had done during labor, but they really couldn't touch the pain of a seven-pound baby coming down your birth canal.

I spent the last few hours of labor in the bath tub. The nurses had pretty much left Todd and me alone and we worked together at getting through the contractions. If my memory serves me well, the contractions were coming every couple of minutes and lasted maybe twenty or thirty seconds?! Todd treated them like a cycling interval… counting down from twenty to one for the interval, followed by rest. Then he would psych me up for the next one. It was awesome—the perfect thing for me. Something I could identify with and understand.

At 5:15 p.m. on June 26, 2008, Alexis Claire Johnson was born. She tore a large hole in my labia that had to be sewn up immediately, with no anesthesia. But we had done it—Todd and I had had the most amazing birth experience. It was the perfect end to an overall won-derful pregnancy. And honestly, I expected nothing less for myself. This was the way things had always been for me. If I focused, worked hard and had passion for what I was doing, I was successful. Period.

Once we got Lexi into our room in the hospital she started crying. No, wait—not just crying—screaming bloody fucking murder at the top on her lungs…and she didn't stop for nearly three months.

Those first forty-eight hours in the hospital were hell. She cried and cried and cried. The nurses were absolutely no help. We had no idea what was going on. She seemed to be nursing, but I really didn't know what that meant. She sucked on my breast, yes, but I never re-ally felt anything. Lots of women say there is this feeling they have called "letting down" when the breast milk releases. I never had that. Ever.

When we brought Lexi home, it was more of the same. She cried and cried. She wasn't gaining weight quickly enough so I consulted lactation specialists at three different clinics or hospitals. They gave me lots of ideas about how to get her to eat. I took herbs and started supplementing my breast milk with formula and hoping, praying that once she ate, she would shut the hell up.

After about four weeks I gave up on breast-feeding and decided to just try and pump my breast milk. If you have not seen a breast-pump machine, it's this awful, horrible contraption that sucks your boob in and out, spraying milk into a tube that drains into a bottle. It is the most unnatural thing. BUT I am from Boulder, Colorado and here we will do ANYTHING to feed our babies proper breast milk!

I did that for about four more weeks, eight hours a day. I read books while pumping, though I couldn't tell you which ones. I was a breast-pumping zombie. I wasn't sleeping, Lexi wasn't sleeping and Todd wasn't sleeping. It was absolutely horrible—I was so depressed. Each morning when I woke up, I had to make a conscious choice to get up and face the day. It was incredibly hard just to get out of bed. I didn't want to face the struggle of parenting—I wanted my old life back. Todd was working a lot and traveling as well. I was petrified of being alone with Lexi. I never thought about hurting her during all of this, but I was miserable. I thought babies were supposed to sleep, be cute and loving. Lexi was none of these things. I remember once coming back from a walk around the neighborhood and I could hear her crying from the end of our cul-de-sac—it felt like I was walking up to the Amityville horror house. Unlike the idiots in the movie, I did not want to stay.

Lexi cried all the time and when she wasn't crying, she wasn't really happy either. I had bought all of these things to make her baby life so joyful, but she hated everything…the Baby Bjorn, the car seat, the swing, the bouncy seat. She just sat there, wide-eyed and miserable. Like she was saying "I want to get back in the womb. I am so over this." I hated taking her to the doctor for her weekly and monthly visits because she screamed in the car seat all the way there. We didn't go anywhere, except those appointments, for months.

At one of my checkups when Lexi was about six weeks old, my OB noticed I was having a tough time and suggested I try Zoloft, an antidepressant. She wrote me a prescription right then and there without any real psychological testing. I thought to myself, holy crap, I am really messed up—but drugs? Antidepressants? For me, that can't be. Antidepressants are for people who can't deal with their own problems. They are a cop-out, and that isn't for me.

Of course, six years later I would swallow those words followed by a shot of humble.

But, at that time, this was what I believed. So I decided to take a friend's recommendation and start seeing a counselor instead. This was the beginning of one of the most important relationships I would develop over the next ten years. My therapist, Jen Sutton, was fresh out of school at that time and had a low-budget office in Boulder that suited me just fine. She was in the basement of a 1950s style office building that clearly hadn't been renovated, ever. Her office was small, probably ten feet by ten feet, with gray carpet on the walls. Yes, the walls and the floor. Luckily for her I was so desperate at the time, I didn't care what her office looked like.

We really hit it off and I loved our time together. I went once a week for months as I sorted out what it meant to be a mom and how to deal with the new challenges I was facing. I had to realize that my life would never, ever be the same. And, let me tell you, I was so pissed about that. I had no idea how hard being a parent would be, but Jen was my sounding board. She didn't judge me, and I found I could tell her anything. She helped me work out my feelings and gave me coping strategies that I still use today. We talked straight talk, no touchy-feely stuff. Jen helped me help myself, pulling things out of me that I didn't know were there. She was my guide and became one of my rocks for years to come.

Jen, my therapist:

When I met you, I remember thinking it would be neat to work with you because you already had a lot of insight and awareness. But

I did wonder how open you would be. You were very clear that first day, you said, I WANT RESULTS, which was a little scary. But as we worked together you always came in with a plan. You knew what you wanted to talk about so there was always a spring board for movement. Plus, we really had a synergy, an alchemical connection that helped us in your quest for growth.

You told me that first day you "lost your identity" the day Lexi was born and that will be a theme throughout the next decade. You always wanted what you HAD rather than accepting what you HAVE. You were always looking for the unattainable. The work we had to do in the beginning of our time together becomes a theme that will continue for many years: the ability to accept.

My therapeutic approach is one of transpersonal psychology, which is the interface between psychology (rooted in Cognitive Behavioral therapy) and spirituality. Basically, it is a holistic approach. I look at "all" of someone, not just what they show up with on the day of their appointment. There are many layers and outside factors that bring someone to therapy and I want to honor all of them. I try to help individuals understand how they think about a situation affects how they feel and then, in turn, directs behavior. How they perceive something will be the biggest factor regarding how they move forward. For you, we had to start at the very beginning and work our way through this process.

About two months after Lexi was born she was officially diagnosed with acid reflux and began treatment. We had to give her a little syringe of medicine every day and voilà, within another month or so she started sleeping and eating better. I was so relieved to have some sort of routine to hold on to. She still cried most afternoons and evenings, but it was at least a little better. During the late-day tantrums we had to do whatever worked to sooth her.

And what I did eventually led to surgery number one...

The only sure bet for keeping Lexi happy was bouncing her on a yoga ball. You know that giant blow up bouncy ball that no one ever uses in yoga? I would hold her close to my chest with my left hand around her back and my right hand under her bottom. She would curl up there and sleep or just be still. I would often try and transport her from the yoga ball to her crib. But when I did, more often than not, as soon as I would take my hand away..."WAAAAAA!!!!" I would have to pick her back up, start bouncing and begin the whole routine all over again. It was like *Groundhog Day* without the groundhog or Bill Murray—it was just me. My quads bouncing up and down in the dark, exhausted, miserable and annoyed by the sweat dripping down my butt crack, hoping and quite literally praying for her to just go the hell to sleep.

CHAPTER 4

So It Begins

ONE THING I have always been good at is suffering. In the early 2000s I could suffer on the mountain bike or on an adventure race with no problem. In the Primal Quest Adventure Race in 2001, I went twenty-six miles on foot over rocky, loose terrain and then rode eighty miles on my mountain bike with a fractured ankle! Once I finally dropped out of the race I was delirious with pain. The race support crew dropped me off at the entrance of a local hotel at 3 a.m. with nothing but the clothes on my back and a bag full of race gear. The manager kindly let me into a room where I proceeded to throw up all night, heaving my guts out in the bathroom from the intensity of the experience. Then in the morning I had to walk to the local urgent care because I had no one to drive me and no money. Insane.

When it came to suffering I was a champ! Until, of course, I had Lexi. Having a colicky baby brought new meaning to the word suffering. When I was pushing my body to its limit in a race, I could dig deep, knowing at the end of the event all of the suffering would be over, followed by the complete euphoria of the accomplishment. Races have beginnings, middles and ends. Every. Single. Time. Having a child that won't stop crying—that seemed to never end.

Lexi was predictably impossible those first few months and all of the things I had read about making *The Happiest Baby on the Block* were totally useless. The advice from the book wasn't working. All the brightly colored, light up, keep your baby busy, plastic stimulation toys were a farce. I felt like I had no control over what was happening and this would prove to be just the beginning.

I used my right hand to support Lexi's body during the yoga ball bounce sessions. The pressure on that hand had caused a condition called Dequervain's Tendonitis. My wrist became swollen and very uncomfortable. It was essentially an overuse injury. Let me say that again, AN OVERUSE injury from bouncing my baby on a yoga ball! How is that even a thing? This is a true testament to the ridiculousness of my life at the time. I would venture to say that I bounced about six or more hours a day on that ball. *A day!* If you ran for six hours a day you would probably end up with an overuse injury. If you lifted weights for six hours a day you would probably end up with an overuse injury. I mean it made some sense logically, but in reality, it seemed so impossibly absurd. But I couldn't use my hand to do everyday things like pour coffee, pick up a pot to cook pasta or turn the key in the ignition in my car without it really hurting.

I tried to be positive as a I prepared to investigate what I needed to do to get better. I am left-handed so it wasn't too hard to imagine being without my right hand for a few weeks. But even though my daughter was only about a year old at the time, I decided I had to do something about this injury.

Having one surgery is not a big deal. And at that point in my life I was grateful that I had never had to contemplate the idea before. I went to see an orthopedist at Boulder Bone and Joint. The same guy had performed a surgery on my husband's wrist a few years earlier. Todd had great results, so I felt safe in his care.

The surgery was just a few minutes long. Though I was sedated, it was outpatient and recovery was only about six weeks. Everything went off without a hitch. But what I hadn't expected was how hard life would be without the use of my right hand. Having one hand with a one-year-old was a recipe for disaster. It was hard for me to pick her up, much less accomplish anything while holding her. I wore the Baby Bjorn a lot to carry her and we got through it. Because I had never really had anything happen to me before, I was calm through the process, and honestly, I don't remember it being that hard. Just a bump in the road.

What would dawn on me much later is the fact that for Lexi, this would be the beginning of a childhood that would require an increased need for self-sufficiency. She had to learn patience quickly. When mom only has one hand, she can't do everything in a timely manner. She might not even be able to do it at all. Lexi watched me suffer through working and managing our house and family with a non-functioning limb, which at the time was short-lived. But this would be a recurring theme throughout her young life. And it breaks my heart just a little writing this…knowing how difficult it must have been for her. The proverbial "they" always say children are resilient and durable. But they are also fragile, impressionable and needy. They need their mothers to be present, secure and available.

Shortly after recovering from the wrist surgery I began running and rock climbing again. My daughter was settling in to a routine and had become a lovely little girl. Our family was doing well and we had moved into a bigger house with the intention of growing our little brood. Since I was an only child I thought that having just one son or daughter would be enough for me. I didn't think I would want more than one, and boy, was I wrong. As hard as Lexi was as a baby, I loved being a mom. I loved it more than anything I had ever experienced. The idea that Todd and I had made this little creature who was curious, energetic and (eventually) happy was just mind-blowing. I wanted at least one more child, and who knows, maybe even three! Since I got pregnant so quickly with Lexi, we figured that having another baby would be no problem. The question was just when we would be "ready." The new house was the first step.

Getting my body back after pregnancy was a glorious thing. It didn't take long for my runs around the neighborhood to turn into jaunts in the Boulder foothills. Even though rock climbing mostly consisted of indoor gym climbing now, I was doing it a few days a week, getting stronger and climbing harder than I had in many years. All in all, things were good...until they weren't.

It started with what I would describe as a cramp in my side. It happened frequently while I was running and sometimes when I was just sitting around. I couldn't really find any rhyme or reason for the pain. It didn't seem to matter if I ate or not, or if I was active or not. Sometimes the stabbing pain would come on without any prompting. Sometimes I would have to just stop whatever I was doing to wait it out.

It didn't take long to go through the battery of tests orchestrated by my family practice doctor and ultimately find out that my gall bladder was not functioning correctly and needed to be removed. I found a great general surgeon at my local hospital that was, shall we say, experienced at removing gall bladders. He was a riot—I loved this guy. He was, in what he would describe as his previous life, a sales representative in the outdoor industry. He had sold snowboards and loved to talk of the good old days when his job and life had been fun. I got such a kick out of his approach to the surgery. He basically said that gall bladders were what kept him in business. Seventy percent of his surgeries were gall bladder removals. So, in other words, this is an organ that humans just don't need, like the spleen or appendix. Apparently, they malfunctioned quite often, so no big deal, just another little surgery.

The gall bladder surgery had zero complications. And I honestly don't even remember if it was outpatient (but I think so). It was about six to eight weeks of recovery before I was back in action. Again, after a few months I felt pretty good and began to run, ride and climb again. Then I got my first introduction to pain that DID NOT have to do with birthing a child.

It was like another cramp, but this time it was down low on my left side, slightly above my pubic bone. Again, I went to see my family doctor who proceeded to order some tests to be done by an OB-GYN. I had an ultrasound and it was determined that I must have had an ovarian cyst. And that the cyst had burst.

One of the many things I have learned living a decade in our broken health care system is that doctors do not do well when they don't have answers. They are often desperate, for themselves or for their patients, to help find out what is wrong. In my case, I was in debilitating pain, and then I wasn't. It would come and go a lot, like the gall bladder pain, but way worse. My family practice doctor and the OB really had no idea what was happening. The cyst diagnosis was a stop-gap that seemed like the perfect little box for the symptoms I had shared with them. Even though there was no actual proof that a cyst had ever existed.

They wanted to give me an answer—it didn't matter if it was true. It was easy. These doctors are forced to see patients every fifteen or twenty minutes all day long. That is anywhere from twenty-one to thirty-two people with health problems every single day. How is it possible to give any of them good care? Even if the doctors want to. How can they really understand the nature of a complex problem in such a short period of time? Many times, they can't. But they have no choice. Medical offices churn patients in and out all day in the name of profits. Never mind that people will get misdiagnosed or not treated at all. I came back to the same office on three different occasions for this pain, and each time they sent me away with nothing except a bogus cyst diagnosis. The pain I was feeling didn't fit into a category like strep throat or the flu, so I was just passed over and moved along. And this isn't a surprise considering how little time they spent with me.

But I wanted to believe them—I mean, they were doctors, right?

So, I did. Any pain I was feeling now was residual from the actual bursting of said cyst. Okay, I thought, sure, that works for me. I should get better any day now.

Then two weeks later I found myself in the emergency room.

It was like any other Sunday afternoon in our little town. Todd and I packed up some water bottles and our little girl for a walk to downtown Louisville for coffee and a trip to the park. Lexi was such an energetic kid, every weekend day included day trips to the playground. Colorado's weather is quite beautiful most of the year so we spent as much time as we could outside. I can remember being at one of the local parks watching Lexi spin in one of those little buckets trying to make herself dizzy when the pain hit harder than ever before. It felt as if my organs were twisting together, tying in knots. It was excruciating. I doubled over the park's woodchips and put my hand down on a concrete platform to steady myself. It was all I could do to stay conscious and focus on not falling over. I thought "this is not normal, this can't be right." And then as fast as it had come it went away, leaving a faint burning feeling in my abdomen. I had to collect myself and try not to give too much away, not wanting to worry Todd or Lexi. Todd was leaving on a work trip the following day and I did not want to alarm him in any way. "Maybe I just have to poop or something," I thought, and then proceeded to go about my day.

On Monday morning my parents had agreed to watch Lexi for a few hours so I could get some work done. Unfortunately, the pain had returned, though not as bad as the day before. Now it was just a dull burning, but I had a fever of 103. Am I sick? I didn't feel sick—no runny nose, no watery eyes, no headache or chills. Just this high fever. Could this be from the cyst? After a few hours I finally decided to go over to my parent's house. I could tell something was wrong, but I just hoped I would get better. I didn't want to be alone and when I arrived I immediately sat motionless on the couch, my head against the hand rest, feet sprawled across the sofa. The pain escalated in my gut as my fever continued to rise. And then it hit me all at once: shit, I need to go to hospital!

When you have gone thirty-six years without ever going to the emergency room, it is quite a disruption to that belief in control.

I was an athlete.

I was healthy.

I had a normal body weight.

I generally felt good, like all the time.

I hardly ever got sick.

I can't possibly belong in a hospital.

Nonetheless, I drove myself there writhing in pain, wanting my mom and dad to stay with Lexi. I figured I would be back soon. I mean, what could possibly be wrong with me?

Avista Hospital, a tiny medical facility in Louisville, has a very quiet emergency room and kind-faced nurses who probably don't see all that much action. But when I walked through that door and complained of stomach pain, I must have looked horrendous because I was admitted immediately. I called my mom and asked my dad to come over. I was certifiably scared at this point. Doctors and nurses were swarming around me, asking me questions while the pain kept growing. I just wanted someone to be there with me to hold my hand. The pain was so fierce I had started slipping in and out of consciousness. The first order of business was to get an IV inserted so they could get both my fever and pain under control. But this would prove to be more difficult than anyone expected.

I lay on the hard hospital bed waiting for the nurses to come in and insert the needle. I was out of my mind in pain. It felt like there were a thousand tiny knives cutting away inside my abdomen. I was desperate for pain relief...but it turned out that I would feel way more pain before I would feel less.

Those nurses that don't see much action, well apparently, they hadn't inserted a lot of IVs either. I was poked eight times before they would actually get the IV in my arm. EIGHT TIMES. It took three nurses before one of them got it. This probably doesn't seem like a big deal, but I remember it like it was yesterday. I felt completely out of control. I could do nothing to help myself. And this was completely new to me—I was great at taking care of myself. But now it was like I was watching a movie, but instead of just watching the plot unfold, I could feel what the character was feeling. I was helpless, miserable and desperate. But when I reached out for help, no one could make the pain stop. It was like a Saturday Night Live skit, but it wasn't funny. What was wrong with these nurses? What was wrong with me? Why was this so hard?? They blamed it on dehydration from the fever. They said my veins were "rolly"—is that even a thing?

Regardless, I eventually received an IV and was immediately given morphine to help control the pain. They must have given me a good dose, because I remember quickly fading into a blissful state of ambivalence. I couldn't feel anything anymore, and that was just fine. I became calm, lethargic and sleepy. Soon I would be wheeled off for a CT scan of my abdomen and a blood draw to determine the cause of the pain and fever. I had never had a CT scan before (this would be the first of thirteen or so scans in the coming years) and I was a bit nervous, but mostly I just wanted answers.

It made me very uncomfortable to not have control of this situation. I have always pushed the boundaries of my limits, but never past them. I remember in college when my girlfriends and I used to travel to Grateful Dead and Phish shows. My friends and I were certainly experimental, but I was often the silent orchestrator. I never let myself get out of control. I dabbled with drugs on more than a few occasions, but I was always riding the line of sobriety and oblivion, never falling into the latter. I always knew where the car was, where we were going and was often the one making sure all my friends were taken care of.

I also love what many people would call "adventure" sports. Rock climbing, mountain biking and trail running were my favorites. But my climbing mostly took place in a gym or outside sport climbing (short, gymnastic style routes with great protection) because, truth be told, I am actually quite scared of heights. I didn't like being 400 feet up on a rock face with only two choices—go up or go down. I didn't feel like I could control the environment around me. I couldn't escape quickly. It made me feel so small, and I hated that feeling. The same goes for water sports—I can't control the water and because of that I don't like being in it. Water can be relentless. White water kayaking and surfing terrify me. Water lives, moves and breathes. I can't manipulate it to fit my needs or abilities, and I don't like that, not one bit.

So, for me to be in this hospital bed waiting for a diagnosis was awful. What was wrong with me? Would I be okay? The morphine helped silence those voices in my head, but they were still there, whispering somewhere in the dark recesses of my mind. *What if something was really wrong? Who would take care of Lexi and Todd? Who would take care of me?*

CHAPTER 5

Diver-tic-u-what-the-fuck

MY WHITE BLOOD cell count was through the roof so the hospital staff deduced that I had some form of infection. In addition, the CT scan determined I had a condition called diverticulitis, which meant there were pockets in my colon where something—presumably waste—got stuck and had become infected. GROSS, right? I was to be admitted to the hospital and would stay there for five days.

This disease is a condition that is often associated with several risk factors, including, but not limited to, obesity, poor diet, lack of physical activity and old age. Presumably this is why I was misdiagnosed on several occasions—I didn't fit into any of those categories, so it seemed almost impossible for this to be true. There was no blueprint for diagnosing a fit, healthy young woman with diverticulitis.

Treatment for the infection would include a massive dose of antibiotics delivered intravenously as well as a liquid diet for several days so my colon could rest and heal. The hospital monitored my white blood cell count until it was stable. I was told if the infection had gotten any worse it would have required a major surgery that may have resulted in my having a colostomy bag (an external pouch that removes waste for disposal through an incision in your abdomen) and a much longer stay in the hospital. So, I was feeling very lucky.

I think the hardest thing about being in the hospital was Lexi visiting me there. It was really hard for her to see her mom lying in a hospital bed, clearly very ill. She didn't want to come up and crawl in bed with me. She could tell I wasn't well and I'm sure it was very scary for her. Today, eight years later, Lexi still talks about the feeling of abandonment she felt during all of those times when I disappeared from the house to stay in the hospital. She was left alone with no mom. Even though I had no choice and this would be the first of many hospital stays…it still feels like a knife in the heart when I hear her say that.

When Lexi was nine years old we decided to take her to a trauma counselor. During one of the sessions she was asked to do a "play" using child therapy props. She was supposed to act out some of the feelings she had during "mom's sicknesses." Watching this unfold was really scary for me—what would she do? And how bad would it hurt?

Lexi took four of those long tubular floating styrofoam things kids use in the pool and set them up like a tepee. She then put a stuffed mama turtle and a baby turtle in the tepee together. The turtles were snuggling when all of a sudden, the mama turtle leaves (Lexi puts the stuffie behind her back) leaving the baby turtle all alone. Without using any words, the baby turtle starts looking around for her mama, but mama is nowhere to be seen. Baby turtle then starts running into the styrofoam tubes trying to get out and find her mama, but she can't get anywhere. Baby turtle stops and then my daughter proceeds to place one-pound weights on top of baby turtle. After she does this, Lexi says "that was how I felt when mom was sick." As you'll find out later, I had to leave Lexi many times to handle my health problems. And even though I felt like I did an incredible job "being there" for her, clearly that isn't how she felt. After she finished sharing this with myself and the therapist, she turned and looked at me with such sad eyes. I knew it was so very hard for her to even share that with me, because she knew it would hurt me. My daughter is an empath, which is a blessing and a curse. She feels things so deeply that sometimes she can't distinguish her own feelings from those of others. She didn't want me to know how alone she felt because she knew I would be devastated. And she was right. All I could think of was where was Todd or "Gma" and "Papa" …where was the village that helped us all get through that misery? They were there for her. But that didn't matter to Lexi. Lexi felt mom was gone and she was alone.

After Lexi finished the "play" our therapist asked if there was anything that mama turtle wanted to say to baby turtle. And through a river of tears, I told her this: "That mama turtle was so sorry that baby turtle felt so alone, mama turtle thought about her baby all the time. Her baby turtle was the light of her life and the reason on many days that mama turtle even got out of bed." When I finished talking and the acting was over she wrapped me in a bearhug, knocking me over on to the floor. And with tears streaming down my face I said I was sorry, and she said, "I know, I love you, Mom."

After getting my official diverticulitis diagnosis the hospital unleashed its protocol on me. My favorite visit was from the dietitian. Now I don't claim to eat a perfect diet by any means. I love Coke Zero, chocolate, Sour Patch Kids and wine. Not all at the same time, but each on occasion for sure. But when the hospital dietitian sat down and talked to me about maintaining a healthy weight (I was 5' 6" and 125 pounds, not really a problem here), I thought "really, this is your answer to my disease. Eat better? *Really*?!" She talked to me about fiber and fruits and vegetables. It was like a trip back to seventh grade health class. I was a former "professional" athlete. Even with the Sour Patch Kids, I was generally pretty healthy. It was comical, I don't think she said one thing I didn't already know. And here is really what I found most disturbing about the whole situation—I was in the hospital with a colon disease and this was the treatment, eat better, get more exercise?! It didn't feel like a promising approach to long-term treatment. Apparently, people with diverticulosis can keep themselves from getting diverticulitis by following these recommendations, but that was already my lifestyle.

There is a difference between diverticulosis and diverticulitis. So, let's back up a second. According to the International Foundation for Gastrointestinal Disorders website, diverticulosis is the condition of having small pouches protruding from the wall of the colon. These pouches are extremely common among Americans—one out of every ten people over age forty, half of those older than sixty, and two out of three over age eighty have them.

Diverticulosis itself is really not a problem, as the pouches themselves are harmless and rarely cause symptoms. But the situation becomes more serious if the pouches become infected from, for example, stool getting trapped in the pouch. If infection occurs, the condition is called diverticulitis. Diverticulitis is more serious because infection can lead to other problems. Diverticulosis leads to diverticulitis in about one out of five to one out of seven cases.

So, what would that mean for me? I guess I hoped it was a one-time thing. I was just the victim of chance and it wouldn't happen again. I would be more careful and somehow it would all get better. I was wrong.

I neglected to mention earlier that between the gall bladder surgery and the first bout of diverticulitis there was a miscarriage. After much debate my husband and I had decided that we were ready for baby number two. Or as ready as we would ever be. We figured he or she couldn't possibly be worse than baby number one, and I really wanted more children. I just loved motherhood even with all the challenges, highs and lows. I felt that being a mom was the world's greatest gift and I wanted it to keep giving. The miscarriage happened while I was on a business trip in Salt Lake City in August 2010, attending the Outdoor Retailer Trade Show. Luckily my industry is a small one and many friends were also there. At the time, Todd worked for a French Outerwear company so he was also working at "the Show." Before a sales appointment, I had gone to the bathroom and noticed some blood in my underwear. I was also cramping and I just knew something was wrong. I tried hard to be professional and give the sales representative the time he deserved when I just started to cry. "Something's wrong," I told him, "I'm pregnant and I need to go." Of course, he was understanding. I went to find Todd and we headed to the hospital emergency room. The hospital performed an ultrasound on the baby and found there was no heartbeat. Our baby wasn't going to make it and I was devastated. I never even thought of this as a possibility. A miscarriage. Our other pregnancy had gone so smoothly. How could this happen? In retrospect, I realize that was very shortsighted of me as millions of women have miscarriages. And I knew that often it doesn't mean a thing in regard to their future pregnancies. But I felt so defeated and so sad. I stayed in bed for the rest of the trade show and flew home with my head in my hands. I just wanted something to go right for me. I had fought hard to overcome my wrist, gall bladder and colon problems, and I wanted desperately to move on with my life.

CHAPTER 6

"No, you're joking"

I'VE MENTIONED MORE than once that rock climbing was one of my passions. Well, actually, I can safely call it indoor climbing now since that is basically all I've done since Lexi was born. I like to be good at things. I have never been okay with being just "average" or "fine" at something. If I am going to do it, you better believe I'm going to put the time in and be good, if not great, at it. My colon had recovered from the infection and I was really enjoying the Boulder Rock Club at the time. I had been going to this climbing gym almost since it opened. I knew everyone who worked there and frequented the venue for many years. It's still my favorite climbing gym. Every time I climb there even now, it feels like a warm hug.

On one particularly lovely afternoon I was roping up with my dear friend and climbing legend, Bobbi. Bobbi and I had raced bikes together a few years earlier when she was taking some time off climbing to pursue ultra-distance mountain bike racing. After realizing she was way better at climbing, Bobbi was back at it and we were still hanging out and enjoying each other's company. On this day I was working on my gym "project," a 5.12—rock climbs are rated on a scale from 5.0 to 5.15, with 5.15 being the hardest. This wall climbs a vertical section first and then kicks back with a fairly steep overhanging section halfway up. It had tiny finger holds that I really loved and it suited my strengths. The feet were the challenging part. The holds required very precise footwork. I had to really pull in with my feet like they were an additional hand. My toes had to almost wrap around the holds in order for me to keep my body attached to the wall. And to make matters worse, I had to clip the rope into quickdraws as I was climbing (called climbing on lead.) This required me to let go with one hand, pull the rope from between my legs and then clip in to the wall for safety. I had been working this route for a few weeks and was feeling confident that this time it would "go" and I would complete it. Bobbi had me on belay—she was making sure I didn't hit the ground if I fell—and I was ready to do it.

I did the bottom part flawlessly and chalked up as I approached the overhang. I assessed the handholds on the upper section and started to climb. Feeling strong and ready I pulled the first two moves easily. At the crux—the hardest part—I used the full force of my left foot to hold my body to the wall when *POP!* go two ligaments in my ankle. Like, literally, *POP!* You could see them floating above my ankle bone under my skin like tiny little worms. The pain was intense—I thought, holy shit, this is it. My ankle is toast.

As an avid trail runner and adventure racer I have had my share of ankle sprains, fractures and rolls on the dirt. Some had been epic ordeals. Remember that stress fracture in the Primal Quest Adventure Race? You better believe there was some ligament damage there. But nothing yet had compared to this injury. It was clear I would not be walking anytime soon. I could put NO weight on my left foot and quite literally crawled to my phone to call my orthopedic surgeon again and ask if his office could see me right away. I didn't want to go to the emergency room—I knew I needed an orthopedic specialist to review the injury. The second call I made was to my husband who was speechless (which doesn't happen very often). Then he said, "No, you're joking."

At the time I remember being very composed, thinking clearly, "I'm hurt, I need to see an orthopedist, this will need to be fixed." I wasn't even upset. I think I was mostly dumbfounded.

The diverticulitis attacks had also become commonplace. The first one was most certainly the worst, but then came a second, and then a third. Each time I would go to the emergency room (they knew me by then), check in, have a CT scan, get checked into the hospital, receive IV antibiotics, get on a liquid diet, my colon would rest and then I'd get better. The doctors were still trying to figure out what to do about me, but only when I was actually IN the hospital. Every time I was released I became a distant memory—out of sight, out of mind. I didn't know what to do either. I was following the protocol given by the team at the hospital. I think everyone, myself included, was hoping the infections would just stop and go away as fast as they had started.

The ultimate fear was that one of the bouts of diverticulitis would be so bad, it would perforate my colon, spilling the waste contents into my bloodstream which could have dire consequences—even death. But the doctors assured me if I kept catching the infections early enough to be treated that would not happen. But, honestly, what kind of life is that? How could that be a treatment plan? And now I ask myself all these years later, why didn't I demand more? How could I have accepted this completely inadequate protocol? "Just make sure you get here quickly." Really? So we can zap your body with radiation, flood you with antibiotics and then send you on your way for a few weeks until you need to come back? Now, when I think about that situation, it sounds like a lot of money for a hospital and a lot of misery for me. But, back then in the middle of the crisis, I just did what they told me. I didn't question. I trusted those doctors completely.

While sitting at the gym adjusting my afternoon schedule to accommodate the visit to my surgeon, my ankle started swelling and swelling until it was the size of a grapefruit. It took all of five minutes in the doctor's office for him to say that surgery was the best option. I could leave the injury to heal on its own, but the damage to my ligaments was extensive and they would likely continue to give me grief. This would be surgery number three in three years, a pattern that would continue to haunt me for years to come.

Surgery was scheduled for November 10, 2010. Lexi was two-and-a-half years old. The doctor would reattach/rebuild the ligaments I had torn and hopefully give my left ankle a long life. He said I would return to full mobility, but the recovery would be extensive. After surgery I would spend two months in a cast. I would be on crutches but couldn't put any weight on my left foot. After that I would get a walking boot to wear for another six weeks. And beyond the boot I would spend six weeks in physical therapy rehabilitating the soft tissue. All this certainly sounded like it would suck, but I knew I could handle it. I wasn't afraid to focus on what I could do rather than what I could not do. I knew I would get strong in the process, both mentally and physically. As always, I tried to look at the positive, keep my chin up and just keep moving forward.

The surgery was performed at Flatirons Surgery Center in Louisville. I had had the wrist surgery there a few years earlier, so I wasn't nervous about the location or the doctor. I knew what to expect and I knew I would be home a few hours after the surgery was complete. Before the operation, the nurses asked me a series of questions about my medications, supplements, birth control, etc. At the time of this surgery, Todd and I were not using birth control, although we were not having a lot of sex because of the diverticulitis. Because of this fact, I had to take a pregnancy test. I joked with the nurse that if I were pregnant it would likely be the second coming because sex just wasn't really happening. After waddling over to pee in the cup, I was relieved to find out that indeed, I was not pregnant. The potential complications of having surgery when you are pregnant are numerous—the drugs, the stress on your body, the energy it takes to recover and sustain recovery—it's all so much to ask of a human being, and even more to ask if that human being is making another life. That doesn't mean it's impossible of course, but when you're thirty-seven years old you need as many positives as you can get on your side if you want to reproduce. And having a surgery during pregnancy is not one of them.

Late afternoon on November 10 I was discharged from the surgery center with a newly reconstructed ankle. I couldn't feel anything due to the nerve block I was given. This kind of anesthesia basically renders your entire leg numb. It stayed that way all day and well into the night. At one point I distinctly remember waking up in the midst of sleep to some of the worst pain I have ever had. I popped up in bed and woke up Todd, "Help, oh my God, Help, oh my God, it hurts, it hurts so bad," I said. I hadn't taken the doctor's advice to swallow the pain killers before bed. How bad can it be, I thought? Plus, I hated pain killers, Vicodin, Percocet, yuck! No way was I going to take those unless the situation was dire. Well, welcome to DIRE.

My ankle felt like it was being squeezed with a truncate. The pressure was immense, but the sharp pain was equally debilitating. I downed two Percocet and waited desperately for the pain to subside. Soon my head started swimming as the drugs started to take effect. I was grateful for the welcome detachment from my reality followed by the relief of feeling no pain, when just thirty or forty minutes earlier I had been completely miserable. Remarkable. Percocet is a combination of oxycodone and acetaminophen, usually given in the form of 5 milligrams of oxycodone and 325 milligrams of acetaminophen. For the average person, one or two of these little pills more than does the job to relieve post-surgical pain, with the exception of more serious surgeries which require additional doses of extended-relief narcotics, most notably OxyContin. Thankfully, this time I didn't need anything that strong to manage my pain.

This was the first time I had ever taken two narcotic pain killers at one time. What happens to your body when you take these pills? According to the National Society of Anesthesiologists, "opioids attach to proteins called opioid receptors on nerve cells in the brain, spinal cord, gut and other parts of the body. When this happens, the opioids block pain messages sent from the body through the spinal cord to the brain." Which, in a nutshell, means you're going to feel a hell of a lot better. The most common side effects of taking opioids are "sleepiness, constipation and nausea." But, because each person is unique, their reaction to taking these drugs is also unique. You can be assured that you won't feel as much (or any) pain, but that may not be worth it, if you can't go to the bathroom or you can't stay awake.

Generally, painkillers made me feel awful and I hated taking them. They had been prescribed to me for both my wrist and gall bladder surgeries, but after taking one or two of them I switched to Advil. It just wasn't worth feeling so out of it and tired. I felt like I was walking around on the moon. I found myself to be unproductive and bloated—two things that generally made me very unhappy.

Of course, I had been given high doses of narcotics in the hospital with the diverticulitis, but that was an extreme situation. I mean I was at a ten on the pain scale. And being sleepy and constipated in the hospital isn't all that big a deal. And quite honestly, who doesn't want to feel that opioid detachment in a hospital? Hospitals suck.

It took only two Percocet to wipe away every bit of discomfort that night and bring me to a blissful state of disregard for what was actually happening to me—my ankle had been rebuilt and it fucking hurt. Over the next week I would take close to twenty Percocet to manage the pain of the surgery. And I couldn't wait to stop taking them. Once Ibuprofen would do the job that was all I took, gleefully throwing out the remains of the prescription in hopes that I would never need to take them again.

After the first week of recovery I started to realize a few things were not quite right, *aside* from the fact that I couldn't walk. My boobs were swollen and I had yet to get my period. Is it late? So much had happened I really didn't know. I wasn't keeping track of these things at the time. I was too wrapped up in the now and dealing with the reality of operating on crutches, managing a house, a two-year-old and a job. Who had time to think about periods! In retrospect, I think it was the boobs that got me thinking, could I be pregnant? *No*, I thought, I mean they gave me a pregnancy test at the hospital and we hadn't had sex since then. And aren't those hospital tests like the most reliable tests ever?? But nevertheless, I needed to double check and make sure I wasn't actually expecting.

I decided that I had put my family through enough in the last couple months, so I would just keep this little concern to myself. I bought a pregnancy test at the grocery store and waited until the "first pee of the morning" to take it, when pregnancy hormone levels are at a twenty-four hour high. Pee on the stick and one minute later your future changes forever. It's that simple—that double pink line is an eternal game changer. For some it's what they are yearning for, waiting months to see it, and for others, it's a devastating reality they hadn't planned for. Either way, it will alter any woman's story forever.

Did I want to be pregnant? Would I be happy if I was? What would it mean for a baby to go through surgery with me, take all those drugs with me? The thoughts were so scary. There was no way to know the future or the impact of past decisions. Just get it done, I thought. I followed the directions meticulously. Pee a little into the toilet and then on the stick for fifteen seconds. Turn the stick upside-down and watch it soak in. Lay the stick on a flat surface and wait one minute for the result. I can't remember what I did for that one minute, but I didn't watch. I walked out of the room and came back to find that indeed, I was pregnant. And had obviously been pregnant during the surgery.

I was mortified. Horrified. I had now had three surgeries, one miscarriage and been hospitalized three times in less than three years. I was *not* ready for this. I wasn't ready for another baby now. And a baby that I had put through surgery…why, why, why was all I could think, why now? Overcome with emotion and literally sick to my stomach, I called downstairs to Todd who was making breakfast for Lexi. "You are not going to believe this," I said. He came to the bottom of the stairs and I was at the top. When he looked up at me, I literally threw the pregnancy test at him. "I'm pregnant."

CHAPTER 7

Pregnancy, Allergies and Emergency Rooms

IT TOOK A few days to settle into the idea of preparing to have another baby. I told my mom, dad and my closest friends. In retrospect I think everyone was worried, including me, but I thought, well maybe this is my "reward" for enduring such misery over that last few years. I've always been, and still am, a believer in fate, in a plan that connects the universe together. Some people call it God or Allah, others look to Goddesses or Mother Nature to find this link. None of that matters to me, I believe that our lives play out exactly as they are meant to. I think we human beings are given gifts throughout our lives to help us grow and change. We can use everything that happens to us to better our lives and the lives of others. So, in this moment, I chose to view this pregnancy as a gift, however ill-timed. I was excited to be a mom again and give Lexi a brother or sister. A little person to make our family bigger, brighter and more dynamic. Todd and I would lay in bed much like we did before I had Lexi and talk about whether it was a boy or girl. What would we name him or her? And what kind of child would he or she be? So many exciting questions begging to be answered.

My ankle recovery was going well, although it was extremely challenging to be on crutches during the Christmas season, pregnant and working industry trade shows. I did the best I could and continued to remain positive. I even crutched around the mall carrying bags of gifts and to make an amazing Christmas for our little angel. Picture it, a thirty-seven-year-old woman clanking around on crutches from store to store holding gift bags in each hand. I even threw some over my shoulders like a backpack. It was certainly a challenge, but I love a challenge. Everything was moving forward nicely until diverticulitis reared its ugly head yet again.

This, of course, was my biggest unspoken fear. I had been hospitalized three times for these attacks and no one could really tell me if they would keep happening or how to prevent them. When I found myself at the Avista Hospital Emergency Room for the fourth time in December 2010 I was mortified and scared. Not just for me, but for the little life growing inside me. I was pregnant with a baby that had already been through one surgery. This time the doctors decided to skip the prerequisite CT scan and just treat the infection. However, they could not use the same antibiotic that had worked for the previous bouts of the disease because it was deemed unsafe for pregnant women. Instead, they would use a drug called clindamycin, an alternative they believed would get the same outcome without harming the baby. The doctors also decided that this time, I would likely do better recovering at home. So, they sent me on my way with a prescription and told me to maintain a liquid diet for a few days, followed by low-fiber food as the pain subsided. Armed with my marching orders, I went home and lay on the couch, waited and hoped beyond hope that I would get through this, and our baby would too.

When you face a situation that seems impossible, sometimes you must just put your head down and move forward. That is exactly what I did that day. I had absolutely no choice. If I didn't treat the infection, I could die. It was really that simple. Our baby was barely seven weeks along and I could not afford to consider what this attack would mean for him or her. I just couldn't. It was almost irrelevant. There was only one choice—take the drugs and pray.

Within eight hours of the first dose I knew something was very wrong. My stomach churned with nausea that seemed completely unrelated to the pain of diverticulitis. This new pain was located much higher, right under my breastbone. I was dizzy and lightheaded. And then without much warning, my body just unleashed. I stood up to run to the bathroom when I just started vomiting on the floor, defecating on the couch. I doubled over in shock. Fear coursed through every vein. The amount of fluid I lost seemed insurmountable. I couldn't control any of my bodily functions. I crawled to the bathroom floor writhing in agony while Todd called the hospital to figure out what was going on. It turns out I was allergic to the antibiotic clindamycin and needed to stop taking it as soon as possible.

When I think back to this time, what hurts the most is that my daughter bore witness to all of this. She was there for every minute. She saw me throwing up all over the floor and pooping in my pants. She saw Todd incredibly scared, desperate to make it stop. There is no doubt in my mind that she must have been petrified. Watching the human being she loves most in the world, in horrible pain and not being able to do anything about it. She was so little then and if there was one moment I could take back from this journey for her, it's that one. Up until that point, I don't think I have ever felt so out of control, so scared, so desperate, so alone as I did on that day. And on top of everything, knowing that I had a life growing inside me, Lexi's brother or sister. I knew right then in my heart of hearts that our baby wasn't going to make it. And I was devastated.

A week later I suffered a miscarriage for the second time, once again destroying our dreams of having another baby. It wasn't unexpected. We were fairly sure that our fledgling fetus wouldn't be able to survive much less thrive given the circumstances, but I was still heartbroken. Losing a baby is quite possibly the most emotionally painful thing a woman can experience. The feeling of loss is so profound. And in some ways, I think this is even more so when you already have a child. You know what it means to create and make a life. You know the joy, the love, the unconditional acceptance of being a parent. It means loving someone unlike anyone you have ever loved. I wanted so badly to love another person as much as I loved Lexi. I wanted that feeling again and again. But it wasn't meant to be. Going through all of this did make me appreciate having just one child. What if we hadn't had Lexi when we did? What if we never were able to have a child? I found the thought soul crushing. It made me so very grateful to have what I did. Even though Louisville, Colorado is simply a town of family ad nauseum. I knew we were not going to be like every other family in our neighborhood with their two or three kids, but I was determined not to let that matter. I was going to make Lexi love being an only child, just like me. I vowed to give her everything, every opportunity I could. She would feel so much love from Todd and me that she wouldn't need it from anyone else. We would be enough for her. I was sure of it.

After losing the baby, I refocused my attention on rehabbing my ankle and getting better. I spent hours upon hours in the weight room and on the bike trainer. When you are used to moving all of the time, it's hard to stop. I don't care much for the traditional gym or exercise class. I like to move in the woods, on trails or roads in the mountains. So, succumbing to a life at our local recreation center was less than appealing. But I needed somewhere to channel all of my frustration and anger. I was mad. I had moved beyond disappointment and now I was just pissed. I put a lot of energy into one-foot top-roping at the Boulder Rock Club. Basically, I would tie into the rope at the climbing gym and climb the routes with my left foot dangling behind me, essentially using just my arms and right foot to get up to the top of the wall. I could actually climb upper 5.11s—pretty hard stuff—with just one foot which was quite astonishing. I was incredibly strong. But none of this strength really filled my soul. I felt empty inside, and trying to fill my myself up with raw power just wasn't making a difference.

Jen, my counselor, helped me try and reconcile the events of the last two years in my mind. I felt like a storm had developed over my head and was following me. It was a dark cloud bringing sickness and disappointment with me everywhere I went. Jen worked with me to begin the process of finding small joys in my life, helping me to start focusing my attention on the good in my world instead of the bad. She taught me that I was in charge of my mind. That I got to control what was going on up there, not the events happening in my life. If I wanted to stay in the place of misery, that was MY choice. She taught me that it was okay to have sad or mad feelings, but it was my decision what to do with them. I could let them take over my life or I could watch them pass like a freight train. There one minute, gone the next.

We did exercises and worksheets that would aid in shifting my thought patterns from despair and hostility to acceptance and appreciation. Quietly, I began to focus on the positive instead of the negative. And in doing this, I was able to find some peace with what had happened in my life thus far. I reminded myself that this was my belief: God and the universe have a plan for me, and this is it. I could choose to hate it, or a could choose to accept it and see the lessons laid out for me to learn.

In May 2011, just four months after my last diverticulitis attack, it happened again. I had to make another trip to the emergency room and was again admitted to the hospital. But this time, I was NOT leaving without another plan of action. Enough was enough, and it was time to deal with this perpetual problem in a new way. I was not coming back here again under these circumstances. EVER.

My gall bladder surgeon was called in to evaluate my case. I was happy to see a familiar face. And turns out he had a plan to deal with my colon and was super excited to have a more interesting surgery to perform. He explained to me that he was going to remove what the doctors believed was the diseased portion of my colon. The infection kept happening in the same area each time, so if my surgeon took out only this part of my large intestine, he reasoned, there would be no more infections.

The doctor was going to cut a four-inch slice between my belly button and my pubic bone. Then he would essentially reach in and remove eight to ten inches of my colon through this incision. He would then reattach the functional ends together and hopefully my digestion would go on uninterrupted. Easy, right? Yeah, no. But, I knew I had no choice but to have this surgery. At some point the diverticulitis would perforate my colon and I would be in some serious trouble. We set the date for July 11, 2011. The doctor wanted to give me some time to heal from the most recent attack while not pushing the surgery out too far. This of course was a dicey choice considering that infections just kept coming, but fortunately I remained well until the date of the surgery.

This would be my fourth surgery in three years, and my first "serious" incubated, dangerous surgery. I mean this surgeon was messing around with my internal organs. If something went wrong, it was going to go very wrong. I was definitely much more scared than I had been for any of the previous surgeries. I had to be in the hospital for the operation and then five additional days for recovery. The one thing I always liked about being in the hospital was not having to cook and ordering food off the hospital menu. For some reason, in the hospital it feels okay to order cheeseburgers and fries or bacon and eggs for breakfast. It's like room service three times a day! And it feels like you don't have to pay for it! When in truth you pay for every last damn thing in the hospital. Unfortunately, when you have a partial colectomy, you can't eat anything even when you get better. After the surgery I would be on a liquid diet for most of my time there, transitioning slowly to a normal diet after several days at home. Totally lame.

On Thursday July 11 the time had come. Of course, my trusty surgeon assured me everything was going to be fine and I believed him. The surgery took a few hours and during it I was under general anesthesia. I was tubed (meaning they put a breathing tube down my neck during the procedure). And when I woke up in the hospital, the thing I remember most was the pain in my throat, not my abdomen—funny what time does to your memory. I also remember this was the first time I had access to a morphine drip. And I loved my morphine drip. I had this awesome little button I could push every time I wanted to forget what the hell just happened to me and float off into semi-conscious bliss. I used it every single time I could. Fortunately, or unfortunately depending on how you look at it, there was a limit on how much I could use. Sometimes I would push the button and nothing would happen. I wouldn't hear the pleasant BEEP followed by the visible drip into my IV. I wanted to keep pushing that button over and over until I forgot who I was or where I was. At the time, I wanted nothing to do with my life. I wanted to fade away.

Lying in that hospital bed during recovery, one of the other things I remember most was feeling alone. Growing up as an independent only child, I was used to being alone. I had to make my own fun and provide my own entertainment. I competed in individual sports and always had relied on myself for just about everything. And that was totally okay with me. But at that moment, I didn't want to be alone anymore. Even though I was happily married with a few great friends, I felt desperately alone. I had assured everyone that I really didn't need any support, that the surgery wasn't a big deal. But that was such a lie.

Back then, I thought my friends didn't want to hear me complain about how hard things were or how many doctors I had seen. I felt like they listened for a short time and attempted to empathize or at minimum, sympathize. But really, I believed they mostly wanted me to just shut up already and get better. This doesn't mean I thought my friends were bad people. I was just depressing to be around. And not because of a bad attitude, but because my life was complicated and it generally just sucked. I didn't have a lot to talk about that wasn't surrounded by discomfort, hospital visits, surgeries, miscarriages and doctors. I didn't want to burden my social circle with my problems. So, I just stuffed my worries, put my head down and plowed through it all. Hoping that on the other side of this colectomy I would finally be able to move on and find more joy in my life.

If you asked my friends now how well I handled myself back then, they would say I was terrible. Even though I had the perception that

I was burdensome, they indeed wanted to help and wanted to listen more than I gave them credit for. It was me that was unable to reach out and let them in. The real truth lies in that I hated being so sad and so broken. Being hospitalized over and over breaks your spirit. What I had perceived as their standoffishness was really their inability to know what to say or what I needed. I wasn't good at asking for help because I truly believed I didn't need it. I had handled everything in my life alone and pretty successfully. But this time was so different. My friendships were so much more important than I could have ever realized. And for each friend that might have kept me at arms-length during this time, there were half a dozen more that wanted to help, they just didn't know how.

After the colectomy was over and I was in recovery, besides my immediate family, only one friend came to visit me in the hospital. When you read this, it may sound pathetic and horrible. I mean, where were all these great friends I had? But the truth is I told them all *not* to come, I was "fine" and it was "no big deal." My best friend from college and the person who knows me best was the only one who saw through all of my bullshit and came anyway.

I remember feeling so sorry for myself. "Why didn't anyone come visit?" I thought. Didn't they know that even though I said they didn't have to come, that meant I really wanted them to? No, of course they didn't! Most people in their mid-thirties haven't had many friends that have undergone major organ surgery, so they don't necessarily know how to act. And if I said it was no big deal, then why should they assume otherwise?

Life Lesson #1 –
You have people in your life who love you. If you need their support, you have to ask for it.

This lesson was twofold. First, I had to learn that I needed more support than I thought from my village of friends. Life can be such a complicated mess and without the most important people in our lives holding us up, it's that much harder to wade through. Second, I had to learn if I wanted support I needed to ask for it. I had to stuff my pride and my "I can take on anything alone" mentality and open up my heart to those who were willing to fill it up with love and support.

As was customary for me up until this point, recovery was smooth and predictable. When someone pulls eight inches of your colon out of your belly button, it takes a while to bounce back. I remember my tummy being sore for a very long time. It hurt to bend over, cough and laugh which was really disappointing. But one thing you get really good at when health problems plague you is acceptance. Recovery from all surgeries have one thing in common—time. You have to be really patient and self-aware. You cannot, under any circumstances, push too hard or you'll be right back where you started.

CHAPTER 8

Snap, Crackle, Pop

AFTER RECOVERING FROM the colectomy, I enjoyed almost an entire year of good health! During this time, I closed my business, Outdoor Apparel Insights, and joined a new venture called Running Specialty Group. I took a full-time position as the Apparel Merchandise Manager. Located in an upscale part of Denver called Cherry Creek, the business was a partnership between a local business legend and the athletic mall store icon, Finishline. You're probably wondering what would have made me leave my cushy job working for myself and all the freedom I enjoyed. Well to tell you the truth, at this point in my life, I was still yearning for something more, something new, something more interesting. I was unable to see how lucky I was or how good I had it. This opportunity was so exciting—I would be part of the first ever attempt at uniting hundreds of specialty running stores under one corporate umbrella. In order to do this, I would have to purchase similar, but slightly different products, for each of our locations across the US. We started with twenty stores on the east coast and grew to about sixty by the time I quit a year and a half later. It was such a challenging job, and so rewarding as the executive team worked diligently to create something new and special. I love a good entrepreneurial endeavor. And I was all in! I had negotiated a four-day work week with one day at home which I spent with Lexi. She was four years old now and happy spending two days a week at "school," two days a week with G-ma and Papa and one day with me. It was really quite perfect. I never thought I could be happy working in a corporate job, but I was.

Since I was working for a running company and didn't want to be a poser, I thought I would sign up for the Aspen Backcountry Marathon instead of racing my bike. I loved trail running and I had worked in Aspen for years. I knew the area and thought running through the backcountry there would be phenomenal. The race was in August and trails were sure to be dry and lined with wildflowers. It would be an exceptionally beautiful experience. The ligament repair in my ankle was holding up nicely and I felt strong again. It was complete-ly healed and totally bomber. In order to prepare for a backcountry marathon, you have to do a lot of up down on the trail. This race had thousands of vertical feet in the twenty-six miles, so I spent a lot of time hiking up the smaller peaks around Boulder and in the summer, I headed up to the high country for more challenging terrain and higher altitude. In retrospect, I think I was probably over-training from the get-go. I hadn't raced a running race in probably twelve years and even back then, I wasn't overly good at it. But my ego at the time was big and I didn't want to show up at the Aspen race unprepared. I wanted to make sure I raced well and was in the front third of the race at least. And ultimately, if I am honest, I wanted to surprise myself, surprise everyone and be actually competitive.

Athletes can be obsessive people, often addicted to exercise like a smoker to nicotine. And sometimes we can't recognize if we are pushing over the edge or beyond the limits of what would be con-sidered "good" training practices. I have been guilty of this on many occasions. More is not always better...did you hear me? More is not always better. In order to gain strength, you must stress the body and then recover. If you continue to stress the body over and over without giving it a chance to heal, you will become injured. Sometimes that can take the form of a physical injury and other times the injury can be mental or emotional. In my case it was always physical.

I remember the trail run before my first hip injury like it was yesterday. It was the most perfect bluebird day in the Indian Peaks Wilderness, an area just south of Rocky Mountain National Park, that boasts high mountains, streams, alpine lakes and abundant trails. It sees much less traffic (i.e. tourists) than "The Park," which is what makes it so special to Colorado locals. The loop was fourteen miles and would take me up to 12,000 feet above sea level. The trail was rocky and beautiful. I remember feeling my legs churning underneath me, powerful and strong, my breath steady, the air crisp.

There's always a slight sense of adventure when you're that high up in the mountains. Weather can change on a dime and it can be easy to get turned around or lost if clouds roll in and the landmarks are gone, especially if you have never done a particular trail. This would be my longest run to date. It was mid-June and the race was scheduled for late summer, so the mileage was in line with what you would expect for that time of year. I felt great going up. The trail was steep so I couldn't really run, so I power hiked at a strong clip up and over the high point in the loop. I was so proud of how far I had come after four surgeries, and so grateful for the opportunity to be out in the wilderness again.

As the trail turned downhill I had to slow down even more due to the rocky nature of the terrain. There were big boulders to hike over and several water crossings. But it was mesmerizingly beautiful—green grass filled with columbines, asters and Indian paintbrush flowers stretched as far as the eye could see. Mossy rocks and crystal-clear mountain run-off filled the drainages while sunlight reflected off the water, revealing the purity of the day.

Upon completing the run my hip flexors—the muscles that runs down from your hip bones toward your quadricep—were incredibly tight from the effort. I was totally wiped out, but euphoric at the accomplishment of completing the loop. I walked down to a stream by my car and soaked my weary legs in the ice-cold mountain water. Sun on my face and now food in my belly—this was my bliss. In these moments I feel like I am not just alive, but living. Four surgeries, five hospitalizations, two miscarriages, and here I was relishing in the power of my body to heal and my mind to never give up. I beamed with a sense of accomplishment so wide I thought nothing could ever hurt me again.

The next day I should have rested, but instead I decided to go climbing.

Bobbi had invited me to Movement, another climbing gym in Boulder, known for its super steep lead climbing wall. While I was training for the Aspen race, I hadn't actually been climbing very much. Bobbi is one of the strongest female rock climbers I know and though she does not care one bit how hard I can climb, I still wanted to keep up with her. Why? I don't know. I just did. The route we were climbing was steep and required a good deal of effort from my tired legs. Climbing something that is overhung takes much more effort from your whole body. You can't just rely on your hands and arms to keep you on the wall. Once the angle kicked out over my head, I should have just come down. But I didn't. I kept climbing, kept reaching, kept trying so hard. And then *POP!* Just like last time. Excruciating pain enveloped my left hip. Instantly I knew I had done something terrible to myself again. It hurt so bad I couldn't climb another inch. I told Bobbi to lower me and that I was done for the day. Even though it was very painful, this injury was not as dramatic as the ankle—I could walk. I figured I would need to rest, but I didn't think for one second that this would be the beginning of the five worst years of my life. It's quite a journey, so hang on.

PART TWO
DRUGS

CHAPTER **9**

It's Just Another Little Surgery

AFTER TAKING A few days off from running, I assumed my injury would go away. It didn't. I could not run at all, not even a hundred yards. In fact, it hurt just to walk. And after about a month without making any progress, I decided to visit my trusty orthopedic surgeon again. Not only did I trust him because of the success I had experienced before under his care, he also specialized in joint related injuries. I told him what had happened while I was climbing and he said he believed it was an acute injury. He couldn't find anything in my X-ray to show that there was any problem with the joint itself. He said the spacing between my bones looked healthy and perhaps I had torn my labrum.

The labrum is defined as "a piece of fibrocartilage (rubbery tissue) attached to the rim of the socket that helps keep the ball of the hip joint in place. When this cartilage is torn, it is called a labral tear. Labral tears may result from injury, or sometimes as part of the aging process." Basically, what I would learn over time is that this piece of tissue acts somewhat like a gall bladder or appendix, as something that exists in everyone's body but doesn't necessarily need to be there in order for a person to function at a high level. But, at the time, repairing the labrum in elite athletes had become quite fashionable. My orthopedist suggested I contact one of the doctors that specializes in these repairs, Dr. Brian, who was apparently one of the best in the business.

I called Dr. Brian's office immediately only to find out that I would have to wait three months to see him. *Three months!* Clearly, I was not the only one with a potentially torn labrum in the Denver Metro area. At the time three months felt like a lifetime to me, and I was not about to wait that long to get a diagnosis. However, I gave all of my information to the office manager and told her to put me on a cancellation list. I told her I was in a lot of pain and really needed to see someone soon. She obliged. But I didn't feel confident that I was going to get in, so I started to research other doctors that might share this specialty.

The first one I discovered was Dr. Mark, a world-renowned surgeon who had honed his craft at the Stedman Clinic in Vail. Stedman is one of the most prestigious orthopedic facilities in the United States. But honestly, at the time, that seemed like a far drive—two hours from Boulder—for an appointment. I felt like I really needed to find something closer, something faster, something easy.

To this day, I am not exactly sure who pointed me in the direction of University of Colorado Sports Medicine. But that is where I found Dr. Omer. He had only been practicing in the United States for about eight months and had come to Colorado to pursue his passion, "hip preservation." He believed that far too many athletes turned to joint replacement before it was truly needed. He knew there were ways to preserve the hip in order for it to function longer and he had spent his short life's work dedicated to this practice. With longevity on their side, patients could potentially avoid a hip replacement and the inevitable loss of function and performance of the joint. I was only thirty-eight at the time and it was incredibly important for me to be able to continue my athletic pursuits beyond this new injury. The other great thing about Dr. Omer was he could see me right away. Yes, I thought, this was my guy!

At the time of my first appointment, the CU Sports Medicine clinic left a lot to be desired. It was small, dingy and dark. The staff was minimal and unempathetic. There were a few well-regarded surgeons on staff, but all in all, I was not overly impressed until I met my doctor. Meeting with Dr. Omer was like meeting the super model of surgeons. He was so cute, confident and had an immense amount of swag. He was a Red Bull athlete, base jumper, runner and surgeon. I remember thinking, this guy is ridiculously hot AND smart. Lucky me!

After my consultation, Dr. Omer ordered an MRI so he could see the damage in my hip. I told him what my orthopedist thought and he agreed that my injury was likely a labral tear. So off I went to the imaging facility to get the pictures Dr. Omer would need to give me a diagnosis.

One of the things I loved to hate was when a doctor came into the room after I have had an X-Ray or an MRI and he or she proceeds to "show" me what is wrong. The doctor would describe my problem in vivid detail, pointing to various points on the image, scrolling through the MRI footage and "making it clear" why he or she is suggesting I need yet another surgery and how they are going to fix my problem. All the while these doctors must know that I can't see shit in those pictures and have no clue what they are talking about. But, when Dr. Omer did that to me after my MRI, I just smiled and nodded. Oh yes, doctor, I see my hip dysplasia and my labral tear. Oh yes, I see that I don't have good cartilage and of course you can cut me open and fix all of that. Makes perfect sense—where do I sign?

In retrospect, I do honestly believe that Dr. Omer had my best interests in mind. I do believe he thought the surgery would prolong my ability to trail run and live my athletic life. I believe he thought he was going to give me my mobility back.

Surgery was scheduled, ironically, for November 30, 2012, my thirty-ninth birthday. What a present, another surgery! I figured if Dr. Omer could fix my hip problem, that would indeed be the best present ever. The plan was to go in laparoscopically (a minimally invasive procedure) and repair the labrum. While in there, Dr. Omer would also perform a microfracture procedure aimed at jump-starting my body into producing new cartilage. Microfracture is a marrow-stimulating technique used in the hip to treat cartilage defects associated with femoroacetabular impingement, instability, or traumatic hip injury. I honestly did not care what he was going to do in there, I just wanted to get it over with and move on once again. I didn't have the patience for all of this medical stuff.

The one thing about having a doctor fresh from Israel is that I really didn't understand everything he said. I mean, I got the gist—surgery, labrum, microfracture, recovery, physical therapy, get better, six months and I'll be running, etc. To me, that seemed like all I really needed to know. I never questioned whether or not the torn labrum was actually causing my pain. If this hot doctor said I needed his surgery, then I must need it. Period, end of story. I also did not ask a lot of questions about recovery or activity after the surgery was over. I knew I would only be able to bear small amounts of weight on my leg, twenty percent I think it was, for several weeks. As I understood the situation, I would be able to ride my bike right away and that movement was indeed *good* for post-surgical healing. To me that meant I could hop on my bike the day after I got home from the hospital, albeit on the indoor stationary bike, and pedal my little heart out.

In 2020 I sat down for a chat with Dr. Omer, almost eight years since this surgery and I got to learn a lot about his recommendations for me then versus what they would be if I walked into his office today. Back in 2012 the focus was more about attempting to fix the labral tear rather than address my hip dysplasia. According to the Mayo Clinic, "hip dysplasia is the medical term for a hip socket that doesn't fully cover the ball portion of the upper thighbone. In periacetabular osteotomy (PAO), the socket is cut free from the pelvis and then repositioned so that it matches up better with the ball." The common thought almost a decade ago was that forty years old was the cut off age for this procedure. And at thirty-eight, I was just too close to that marker. That's why Dr. Omer didn't push me in this direction. It was a more invasive procedure than the one we had planned and would involve additional months of recovery. He thought, at the time, that we were making the best decision for my future. He still states that he wouldn't change the way he approached my case.

However, if I walked into his office today, he would be more confident that I should actually go the route of a PAO rather than the labral tear and microfracture procedure. But back in 2012, he felt he didn't have the credibility or historical context to make that statement.

Dr. Omer:

In the past five years I have treated a large group of very active women from all over the country. Some of them have been high level Ironman and ultra-distance runners. All of them suffering from similar symptoms, damage in connection with hip dysplasia. Now these cases comprise 95% of my patient load. And the ages range from 45-58. For each of them I performed a PAO and have had 100% success, no exceptions.

So, when did this age shift happen? To be honest, it was slow. I would perform the surgery on someone in their late 30's and then they would come back 5-8 years later at 45 and say, "You mean you're not going to fix my other hip just because of my age?" And I was like, well you have a valid point. Of course, there are other objective criteria to determining a surgical candidate. It is never one size fits all. But, for me, a hip is a hip. When the patient is on the table and I am ready to operate, they are ageless. The parts are still the same.

Of course, the other piece of the puzzle is that today, my techniques are much better and much more refined. And I not only continue to work toward evolving as a surgeon but, also to teach my fellows these proficiencies. If you came to me today, I believe the outcome would have been much different.

I didn't want to lose all of my fitness again. I didn't want to start over again. I just wanted to have the surgery and be okay, quickly. I was terrified of being out of shape, petrified of being soft, flabby and lazy while recovering. I wasn't thinking about the long-term effects of my choices, I just wanted everything to hurry up already—surgery, healing, recovery—so I could get back to my awesome life. But during this time an old demon from young adulthood reared its ugly head. Yes, my life was generally quite charmed, but I wasn't immune to all hardships and struggles. Growing up in competitive gymnastics does have some pitfalls.

I was bulimic.

In my last year of college, I struggled with what would come next. In order to curb my mounting anxiety, I found myself spending a lot of time in the gym working out, running and climbing. In college I danced for a couple of dance companies, but I also smoked a lot of weed and ate a lot of pizza. Let's just say I wasn't the skinniest, but I wasn't really heavy either and I didn't really care. But as graduation loomed, my life felt out of control. I had no idea what I was going to do with my worthless degree in Recreation. In an effort to exert some control over my life, one thing I decided I could control was how much I exercised and ate. And control it I did. But it was a slow burn. I didn't just decide one day I was going to become bulimic.

As I upped the exercise and watched my diet, I started to lose weight. I was getting very fit and often got compliments from people saying things like "wow, you look great; have you lost weight? I wish I looked as good as you," etc. I loved this attention and definitely craved more of it. I started writing down everything I ate, counting every calorie and restricting my eating habits substantially. I measured my cereal, cut pieces of cheese into little bits, bought everything that was labeled light, fat free and diet. I worked out between two to three hours a day eating less than 1,500 calories. I took herbal laxatives, colon cleansing pills and diuretics.

At the time, my behavior mirrored more of an anorexic, but the problem with being anorexic was that I loved food and missed it desperately. The binging and purging started at my job. I was a waitress at a small restaurant in Bloomington, Indiana called Opie Taylors. They specialized in cheap beer, fried food and chili. At the time, I was a vegetarian, so the chili was of no interest, but the fried potatoes, fried zucchini, fried anything, I could not resist. And once my food-deprived body started eating one of those delectable items, I could not stop. I would just stuff my face and with each bite I would feel more horrible about myself. And on more than one occasion, I would be overcome with so much disgust in myself that I would go into the customers' bathroom and make myself throw up. It certainly makes me cringe now, how unbelievably disgusting that was. But back then it seemed perfectly reasonable.

When I reflect back on this time, I do think that our backwards society had something to do with it. The media constantly featured only the skinniest women on magazine covers. Celebrities were always touting fad diets and they were all incredibly thin. I mean, the skinnier I got, the more compliments I got. And when my girlfriends tried to stage an intervention when I was just above 100 pounds (I am 5'6"), I just assumed they were jealous. That is pretty frickin' skinny and I am sure I was bordering on gross, but I could not see it at all. On some level, I knew I was doing something awful to my body with the throwing up and the herbal supplements, but I could not seem to stop it.

The situation finally came to a head at my home in St. Louis during one of my trips back to visit my parents over the summer. I'm sure my mom knew something was wrong with me, but didn't know exactly what. She was watching me closely though. And one afternoon her 100-pound daughter decided to make chocolate chip cookies and proceeded to eat almost half the dough before even one cookie could be baked. Once I had one bite of the batter it was all over for me—my will power evaporated and down the hatch went a pound of cookie dough. I was mortified at my behavior and felt compelled right then to expel the food from my body as quickly as possible, so I went down to our basement bathroom and threw up. Little did I know, my mom had followed me and witnessed the atrocious act for herself.

My Mom:

She wouldn't look me in the eye. She had acted happy and relaxed since she got home but she wouldn't lock eyes with me. I wasn't sure what was wrong, if anything, but there's a gut feeling that nags at you when you love a child. I struggled to follow her that day...If I don't go down the stairs to check I won't have to deal. I didn't want to know...I didn't want to do this. The hardest thing I ever did was open the bathroom door. I suspected, I knew. Dear God. I was horrified at what I saw; red watery eyes, beads of sweat on her flushed face, wiping her mouth with the back of her hand. Guilt all over her face. The rest was a blur of tears and angst. Later, I remember worrying that this would be a battle she might have to fight for the rest of her life...or that she could lose her life. It was terrifying.

I think if you asked my mom today she would tell you this was one of her lowest, most painful moments as a parent, when she questioned everything about the choices she had made for me and what she could have done to prevent this from happening. I honestly don't know if there was anything she could have done. It's hard to say. I grew up in a sport that was very body-conscious and I had been told on more than one occasion that I was too heavy to be an Olympic-level gymnast. Weight and body image were always at the forefront of my mind as a child and I don't think anything could have changed that. I put such a high value on body image and other people's perception of me. I wanted people to think I was amazing, pretty, fit and awesome. But inside at the time, I didn't feel like any of those things were true. I was confused and lost, not knowing where I was going or what value I had as a human being in the world.

After my mom caught me purging, I never did it again. I certainly thought about it more than once, but I think seeing my mom so devastated was actually really scary for me. I realized how perverse my behavior had been and that I was only hurting myself. Another big step in moving on from this behavior was going on my National Outdoor Leadership School Semester. I left for the trip just a month after that faithful day at home. Living in the "wild" simplifies everything—there were no mirrors, no place for me to place judgment on myself. We had just enough food to power our various journeys, so binging and purging were not exactly options. I found a sense of peace out in the wilderness. And even though I was able to take some of that back home to my life in Indiana, I don't think I was completely cured of my toxic thought process. I still fight it to this day.

One of the first things that went through my mind whenever I had an injury or needed a surgery was I can't exercise, therefore I can't eat. That thought still plagues me to this day. It's there before I can even recognize its toxicity. The difference now is that I can catch it and then reshape its relevance. Instead of thinking crap, now I'm going to get fat because I have to have surgery, I think, I need to make better, healthier food choices while I'm healing. I focus on the need to take good care of my healing body rather than depriving it from the nutrition it needs to get better by restricting my calorie intake to nil. But sadly, back in 2012, I was not quite there yet.

The first thing I wanted to do after my surgery with Dr. Omer was get on my bike. I mean, he did say "movement would be good for healing." However, he did not say—or at least I don't remember him saying—that I should not use any resistance. I'm pretty sure within twenty-four to forty-eight hours of my operation I was on my trainer in the basement riding too hard with too much resistance. I was so worried about losing my fitness and ultimately getting soft that my sole focus was not on recovering, but on maintaining my body image and strength. What an idiot I was! It almost makes me angry now to write this. How pathetic. How shallow. How short-sighted. How could I not have seen the need to rest, to allow my body time to heal? I mean, I had been through four surgeries already and I *had* learned the value of time and the need to give the body space to heal. How could I have reverted back so quickly to my old ways? How could I have cared so much about how I looked and how athletic I was? How could I place so much value on something so insignificant? My ego was so big and my obsession with fitness so profound. It was my identity. I believed it was something I could control. The reality was, I clearly hadn't learned a thing in the past four years.

At my post-op appointment about a week after the surgery, I clearly remember Dr. Omer waltzing into the office and literally hopping on to the patient table and saying—and I quote—"Man, your hip was fucked." Now, that was a first.

He proceeded to tell me in his broken English about the surgery and what he had done to fix my issues. When I told him I had been riding the trainer, he scolded me for potentially riding too hard. And I pleaded the Fifth, saying I hadn't known I was supposed to ride with no resistance (which I really did believe). I was worried that maybe I had done some damage to his work by overdoing it, but he assured me that was unlikely.

But still, to this day I wonder, what if I had not gotten on the bike that day? What if I hadn't put on my headphones with my angry hip-hop mix and pedaled my little heart out? Would I be writing this?

Because of the surgery I was able to work from home for the better part of three months. I took a few painkillers during the first week post-op, but was quickly able to manage the pain with just Tylenol and ibuprofen. I went to physical therapy and tried to be patient with the healing process. But this was surgery number five, and I was getting tired. Tired of building myself back up from nothing. Tired of being uncomfortable and not living up to my abilities as an athlete.

I needed a goal.

I needed something to work toward. I started perusing the mountain bike ultra-marathon websites and came across a new race called the Hundo 100. It would be held in Bailey, Colorado the following June. That's it, I thought, just what I need, a race! I signed up as soon as the registration opened and set my sights on getting back to racing after five years of motherhood and surgery. I was pumped.

I try to live by what I call the three D's: dedication, discipline, determination. It takes all three of these things in spades to train for a 100-mile bike race, especially if you're starting from quite literally nothing. After my incident on the bike trainer immediately after surgery, I did pull the reins on my efforts to keep my fitness at a certain level. I did focus more on physical therapy and tried to silence the nasty voices in my head telling me I would never get it back. I took six weeks post operation to just exist and heal. And I did get a little soft—but you know what, it didn't matter. I was laser focused on this bike race and nothing was going to keep me from making it to the starting line—nothing.

By January 2013, about two months after the surgery, I was back at it. But this time I didn't have the luxury of the flexible schedule I had known for most of my life. I had a full-time job now and my office was forty miles from my house. How was I going to put in the training to get ready for this race? Hmmm? Time to get creative.

Like any good Type A control freak—I needed a PLAN!

There was a 6:00 a.m. spin class on Tuesdays I liked, check.

There are two days in the weekend and one of them could be a long ride, check.

But what about the rest of the week? My office was too far for me to ride both ways. Solution: Drive to work in the morning with my bike, ride home, ride back to work the next morning, drive home. Perfect. Check.

All I needed was a route to the office, a bike light and a very warm pair of gloves because it was January and the sun was in short supply.

I knew it would take a few tries to figure out how to get there, but I was up for the challenge. I'm always up for a challenge.

Now there's a great bike path that connects Boulder to Denver, but back in 2013 that was still just an idea in someone's head. It would take some serious navigational skill through some dicey areas of Denver with no bike lanes to get to the lovely Cherry Creek paved bike path which would provide the last four miles of concrete before arriving to work.

In retrospect, I think this probably was the most productive stretch of my adult life. I only had a full-time job for about eighteen months, but in that time I accomplished so much. When I took the job, I thought it would be just about impossible to get everything done. But I was wrong. I had a routine—every week looked the same.

Monday – work, rest
Tuesday – spin class, work
Wednesday – drive to work, ride home
Thursday – ride to work, drive home
Friday – home with Lexi
Saturday – Long ride, laundry
Sunday – Medium ride, grocery store

When you completely lose your ability to walk normally even for a short time, every milestone seems monumental. Those first real rides post-surgery were very difficult. There were times in the beginning where I would overestimate the number of miles I could be on my bike. I would struggle just riding up the small rolling hills back to my house, pedaling so slowly I was barely moving. Old men with hairy legs flew by me—it was soul crushing. I could visualize a time when I was fit and fast, but that seemed like a lifetime ago and I wasn't sure I could ever get back to that. I remember calling Todd from my parents' house just three miles from home and having him come pick me up because I couldn't pedal my legs a single revolution more. But regardless of all of the defeats, I never thought once about quitting. It never even crossed my mind. My hip was holding up and I had no pain post-surgery. I knew if I just kept showing up every day and working hard, eventually the tables would turn for me.

Sometimes showing up meant riding to work in the dark when it was twenty degrees. Sometimes it meant riding to work in a snow-storm or home through a vicious evening windstorm. But I just kept going, kept moving forward, believing it would all pay off. And at some point, in the late spring, it did. I got fast, faster than anyone else I was riding with. By April, I was burying men on the Peak-to-Peak highway above Boulder that runs between 7,500-9,500 feet above sea level. I was flying around on my bike and loving it.

I was all business, and wanted this race more than I wanted any-thing else. The last ultra I participated in was in 2007, so it had been six years since I had rolled up to the starting line for this kind of ad-venture. Thankfully, I had prepared enough times, I knew how to get myself there. I knew what kind of preparation was necessary and it was my sole focus.

When June rolled around I was absolutely ready for the race. I taped a piece of paper on the top tube of my bike that said, "4 years, 8 doctors, 5 surgeries, my race, my time." I was super confident in my ability to finish the race and thankful that Todd, my parents and Lexi would all make the trip up to Bailey to cheer me on halfway through the day.

As we rolled out on to the course, the adrenaline started pumping through my body. I was ready for an adventure and a great day on my bike as I settled into my pace and tried to make sure I was eating and drinking enough. The first sixty miles of the race were on single track and there was a lot of congestion on the trail. I just tried to be calm and patient. Ultras are not won or lost with quick moves—I have completed them by being smart with my nutrition and riding MY own pace and not trying to keep up with any one rider. Individual's strengths will ebb and flow throughout the day, and you never re-ally know who's pushing themselves to their limit. I didn't know who would crash or bonk or be unable to continue. I had to ride my race.

Ultimately it was me against the course. Everyone and everything else fell away and I just pedaled.

Ahhh, I felt so great that day! Sure, there were some low points, but I never thought about tapping out. I knew I was going to complete the course and that it would likely be my fastest 100-mile race ever. Turning into the finishing stretch I remember feeling so satisfied. My eyes welled up with tears and I was so grateful for my ability to get to this point. As I crossed the line I hugged my family and repeated over and over "I did it, I really did it!" Eight months ago I couldn't even walk and now I was completing a 100-mile mountain bike race. "Damn, I am awesome," I thought. I was so proud at that moment. So full of life. Nothing could stop me from realizing my dreams—nothing.

The ride earned me third place in my age group and a top six finish overall. Standing up on the podium that day might have been one of the most amazing moments of my life up to that point. I had overcome so much to get there. I was on cloud nine! Unstoppable!

CHAPTER 10

All Good Things Must
Come to an End

IT TOOK SO much for me to get ready for that race. I was so committed and had worked so hard, and honestly once it was over I was
exhausted from the effort. I was tired of riding my bike and started
setting my sights on being able to run again. In fact, I couldn't wait
to run! Dr. Omer said I could return to running six months after the
surgery and it was July. Almost eight months had passed since the
birthday operation.

You would think because I was a "professional" caliber mountain
bike racer that I was in love with cycling. I was not—I was in love
with being great at something. Don't get me wrong, I like riding my
bike, and love where it takes me. I can cover so much ground on a
bike. I mean riding 100 miles in the backcountry is an incredible
gift to the soul. Slipping through Aspen trees with their bright yellow
leaves in the fall or crossing fields of wildflowers in the summer is
amazing. But I don't like navigating the trails with a machine. There
are moments when I feel like my bike and I are one unit moving
through the wild, but there are many more instances when I feel like
the bike is a hinderance to pure movement. If given the choice, I
would much rather cover ground on my feet than on a machine. For
me, that is just a fact. I continued to nurture my cycling because I was

better at mountain bike racing than I was at trail running. I was also much less prone to an overuse injury riding my bike.

Trail running has a sort of primal quality to it. It feels like moving through space as the body was originally intended to move, fast and light over dirt and grass. I love this feeling and there really is no substitute for it. I could not wait to get back into the Boulder foothills running my favorite loops, covering many hours and miles moving efficiently through the woods. So, on July 1, decided it was time to run.

Mountain biking and running are very different sports and being good at one DOES NOT translate to immediately being good at the other. I remember my first jog was a four-mile loop on a very easy trail with virtually no elevation change. You would think if I could ride 100 miles on a mountain bike, I could run four miles without too much trouble. But the truth is, running is just SO different. And those four miles made me very sore. I had a whole new set of muscles to start training and a lot of work to do to get my running fitness up to par. But, hey, I was the queen of the comeback, so this process was nothing new. I thoroughly enjoyed the journey back to running after both my ankle and colectomy surgeries, so I figured this time would be no different—but it was. Very different.

Almost immediately following those first few runs, the pain returned to my hip, and it was much worse than it had been before the surgery. I tried to go slower, to rest longer between jogs, but nothing was making a difference. I didn't want to go back to riding my bike, I wanted to run. And I wanted to run right now. I kept trying, kept lacing up my sneakers and heading out to be ultimately defeated by the pain. The impact associated with the effort of running was just too much for, what appeared to be, my still damaged hip. I was so defeated. And now I was pain again.

Damn it. Damn it. Damn it. Why? Why? Why?

At this point, my God, I was so pissed. I was mad at the situation and mad at Dr. Omer. I felt like he lied to me. He said I would be fine, that he was going to fix me. At least that's what I thought he said through all that broken English. But the truth is, he hadn't. He said, there was a really good chance I would be back to normal in six months. He said I very likely would be able to run again and return to all my activities. Granted, he made no promises, most surgeons don't, but he said he felt really good about it. But this was not good, not good at all.

I started to do what I should have done before I let another doctor cut me open—research. I learned that the surgery I had was very, very new and only a select few doctors in the country were even performing it at all.

Then I started to reflect on some of the red flags that had led up to the surgery itself:

- The "research" surveys I had to fill out. Every time I went to Dr. Omer's office I had to fill out a pain questionnaire pre- and post-op. You know why? Because this surgery was so new doctors really had no clue how people were going to do over time. They were looking to measure their success.
- There was no surgery code for the insurance company to bill. Dr. Omer had to call them directly to get approval. Labral repair had not even hit the insurance market yet.
- I could find almost nothing online about labral repairs.

Now don't get me wrong, Dr. Omer had nothing but the best intentions and he was a good man. But, in 2013 it was clear as day to me that the surgery had not worked and in fact, I felt worse than I had before he cut me open.

Time for a new doctor. I figured the best idea was to attempt to see the ever-famous-yet-oh-so-elusive Dr. Brian again. I called the office and got on the schedule. I went to see him at his office in Denver October, 2013, almost a year after my surgery with Dr. Omer. By then I was uncomfortable pretty much all the time. Dr. Brian, like Dr. Omer, was young, savvy and full of confidence. He waltzed into my room with the same pain questionnaire I had filled out before. Sketchy. But what choice did I really have? I mean according to my first MRI I had a torn labrum (which in theory had been fixed). What would Dr. Brian suggest I do? I had no idea, but I had to give him a chance.

I told him about my surgery with Dr. Omer and how disappointed I was with the outcome. He said before he could make a recommendation, I would need to get another MRI to assess the current situation. And in order to do this, I had to go to "his" special imaging place, conveniently located about an hour from my house. I mean there were probably twenty imaging facilities within twenty miles of where I lived, but NO—I had to go to this one. Okay fine, whatever. He said they would go through a specific protocol there to make sure the labrum was indeed the source of my pain. That sounded promising. So, on October 17, 2013 I went to have my fancy MRI.

When I got there the first thing the technicians did was give me an ultrasound guided injection directly into my labrum, which was quite painful. The purpose of the injection was to numb the labrum. Then they gave me thirty minutes to attempt to aggravate the injury and see if I could still feel the severe pain I had been experiencing. If the labrum was causing my pain and it was numb, I should feel nothing.

Problem was, I could not feel any difference. I could not even tell I had had an injection. I went outside, walked, jogged and sat in the waiting room. It hurt the whole time. The injection did absolutely nothing. I told the MRI tech this information before I crawled into the MRI machine for the images.

When I met with Dr. Brian after the appointment and told him how I experienced no pain relief with the injection, he said, "huh, that's weird."

Then he proceeded to show the MRI images to me. He said that I still had a torn labrum. He believed that sometime post-surgery I had torn it again, maybe running or maybe on that first fateful bike ride on the trainer after the operation. I will never know and either way the outcome was the same. Dr. Omer's surgery had not worked. But

Dr. Brian assured me, I was in luck because he was one of the only surgeons in the country actually reconstructing labrums with cadaver. He never again mentioned the fact that the diagnostic injection performed at the image facility did not prove the labrum was source of my pain. And you know what, neither did I—he brushed it off like some anomaly and I just went along with it. This was such a poor choice. Once again, I blindly put my faith in another doctor who seemed to have all the answers. What I should have done was demand another test to confirm that he was working on the right part of my hip. But I didn't. Dr. Brian was completely booked up at the time, and I knew if I waited any longer the whole process would drag on and on. I just wanted to be better. Even with no more tests, I wouldn't be able to get into surgery until the middle of the following year!

By this time, the pain was constant and got worse when I exercised. I couldn't run, couldn't ride, couldn't sit in my car without being uncomfortable. Pain was everywhere and it was harder and harder to escape it. I asked hardly any questions about this next surgery either. I didn't care what it would take to recover. Facing a sixth surgery in six years, I just wanted it all to be over.

Because of my pain level and my clear misery, Dr. Brian prescribed Vicodin, 5 milligrams of hydrocodone and 325 milligrams of acetaminophen. Up until this time, I had hated painkillers, but I knew I really needed them now. Surgery was scheduled for June 26, 2014—my daughter's sixth birthday. I had a few months to live with the pain and wait.

I treated myself to daily pain relief around 3:00 p.m. I would take two Vicodin and enjoy a few hours of manageable discomfort before bed. Each day, I could not wait until 3:00 p.m. I watched the hours, counted down the minutes. Some days I would give in at 2:00 p.m. and others I could hold out until 4:00 p.m., but it became a daily ritual, one I would continue in one form or another for the next three years.

Pain management is tricky. In all honesty, a couple of Vicodin a day is not the end of the world, and many people use small doses of opioids to manage pain before a surgery. The problem with pain killers though is you build up a tolerance to them. And all of a sudden 10 milligrams of hydrocodone didn't quite cut it anymore, and I needed something stronger to get the same level of relief. After about thirty days on my regiment, I requested and was granted a bigger dose—10 milligrams of hydrocodone and 325 milligrams of acetaminophen per pill. I doubled my daily narcotic intake to 20 milligrams and began to notice something new about my afternoons and evenings. Not only was I not in pain at night, I was much more capable of dealing with my situation then, caring just a little less about what was happening to me. The opioids dulled the sharp edges of my life and helped me find peace with facing another surgery.

I also spent a lot of time in therapy during these months between surgeries. I was seeing Jen once a week or at a minimum bi-monthly. Not only was I suffering in my body, I was also struggling at work. Lexi was about to transition from day care to Kindergarten, and the perfect schedule I had set up with work thus far would no longer be possible. The school day was from 8:00 a.m. until 3:00 p.m.—just seven hours. There was no conceivable way for me to work a full-time job when my daughter only had school for thirty-five hours a week. How would I cover the other five hours plus the commute? As usual I attempted to think outside the box. Okay, I thought, what if Todd takes her in the morning and I leave for work at 5:00 a.m. arriving easily by 6:00 a.m. Then I work straight through lunch until 2:00 p.m. (eight hours); then I leave to come home and pick up Lexi from school. Brilliant! I pitched this to my boss and I could tell immediately he was not psyched. But at the same time, he could not really argue with me. I mean I was agreeing to work the required forty hours and I would likely continue working once I got home and Lexi was settled in with friends or whatever. I had been doing a really good job and I had made some amazing connections. I didn't want to leave, but I also wanted to be an available mother.

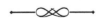

Having just one child is a really unique situation. Most people think it is SO much easier than having multiple children, and I would guess when the siblings are younger that is absolutely the case. But really, they are young for such a short time. When you have an only child, you become not just a mother, you become a sister or brother, a playmate and a best friend. I love the relationship I have with Lexi. We are so close! But that relationship requires constant maintenance. We are always hanging out and doing things together. There is no "go play with your sibling." There is playing with mom or there is playing with no one. Todd was always working.

I didn't want to send Lexi to day care after school. Seven hours was a long day for a six-year-old, and I thought adding more social situations would just be too much for her.

My boss did reluctantly agree to my request for these new hours, but I could tell he did not like it. This request would ultimately be the beginning of the end for me at Running Specialty Group. And that was just fine. Recently, I'd had an incident with Lexi that made it clear I was trying to do too much anyway!

It was the spring before Lexi was heading to her new school, Peak-to-Peak Charter School in Lafayette, Colorado. We chose this school because it was supposed to be one of the best schools not just in Colorado, but in the entire country. The school had sent an email out to all of the incoming Kindergarten class inviting everyone to a picnic. This would be an opportunity for the teachers, kids and parents to meet one another. Well, I did not read the email very closely because apparently, we were supposed to bring blankets and picnic baskets full of food for the event. Well, I showed up with absolutely nothing and Lexi was horrified. I texted Todd and told him he had to leave work immediately and get his ass to the school with food and a blanket like five minutes ago. This was our first real school event and I had totally screwed it up. Not because of actually forgetting of the food or whatever, but because I had become the mother I never wanted to be. I was too busy to read the email. I was too stressed, too overwhelmed and in pain all the time. I did not have the space to handle a school-age kid with school kid needs and my job. It was clear I needed to make a change.

Shortly thereafter, I quit my full-time job and accepted a more flexible position working for Sopris Sales, a sales agency that handled the Rocky Mountain region for the outdoor brands Swix, Lole and Bison Belts. I had been working as a buyer for almost twenty years by this time and I thought perhaps I wanted to sit on the other side of the table and work in sales. And oh man, did I ever suck at that job.

I thought because I had so much experience as a buyer and was generally considered an opinion leader in the outdoor industry that people would be interested in what I had to say. I thought other buyers would be excited to work with me. I thought I was going to be able to help a lot of businesses. But the truth was they didn't want to hear anything I had to say. The buyers came to our showroom with their own ideas and thoughts. Sometimes I agreed with the choices they made and sometimes I didn't, but either way, it didn't matter—they did not care. And I hated that they didn't care what I had to say. Everyone had always cared what I had to say! (I sound like such a baby, I know.) I mean I had been asked to sit on retail advisory panels for The North Face, Marmot, Outdoor Research, Arcteryx, Patagonia, etc. I was so good at buying outdoor/run clothing by this time, I could have done it with my eyes closed.

I quickly realized the job really was not for me, but I loved my boss and she didn't seem to care that I had all of these health problems and was taking a steady stream of Vicodin every afternoon. I still worked hard for her and felt grateful to have employment that was completely flexible. I worked predominantly from home, but had to travel to Denver where our showroom was located frequently, but that was easy, even during school day hours.

My responsibilities were mostly to support the business from the back end. I was basically an office manager. It was super easy and I dealt with running reports and requesting information from brands for retailers. I took care of unpacking season samples and kept the showroom tidy. Piece o' cake, which really helped considering all that I was facing with the daily pain and my impending surgery. As June 26 grew closer, I grew more scared, but I was also hopeful that this was where this journey would end for me and I could get back to a normal life.

Not a chance.

CHAPTER 11

Darkness

WE CELEBRATED LEXI'S birthday early in 2014 and I made sure we had a ton of fun. I didn't want her to feel like the surgery was going to ruin her special day, and quite true to form she was great about it all.

On June 26 I was supposed to check into the hospital around noon which was a couple of hours before my surgery scheduled for 2:00 p.m. The surgery would take place at a hospital solely dedicated to orthopedics. They had built a whole new section just for Dr. Brian's surgeries—he was that good! At least that's what I thought at the time. Now I think, he just brought in that much money.

I do believe Dr. Brian had the best intentions as well. I knew he wanted to help me and would give the surgery his best shot. I think the question that will always remain in my mind is why did he want to still perform a labral reconstruction if the labrum had not proven to be the source of my pain? I had the power to question further, but I did not. I had the power to say NO or to get another opinion. But I didn't. He was "the best," right, world class?! If he thought I could be fixed then why shouldn't I believe him?

Life Lesson #2 – Doctors are human too

Because human beings are not perfect and they make mistakes all the time. Because humans are inherently imperfect. The only person I really have to blame for the choices I made is me. I can't point fingers at any one doctor and be like "it's your fault." It's not. It's mine. I signed the papers, I agreed. I knew there was a chance it wouldn't work, but I didn't care. Some chance was better than no chance, and when you're living with chronic pain, some chance is plenty good enough reason to try.

Growing up I think I believed that if you were a doctor, you knew everything about the human body. If I was sick and the doctor said I had the flu, then I had the flu. I never thought about questioning my doctor, or that, God forbid, he or she might be wrong. But the truth is doctors make mistakes just like everyone else. They misdiagnose. And sometimes, they just don't have the answers their patients are looking for—sometimes they have no answers at all.

I spend a lot of time now talking with people searching for answers in the medical field. I urge everyone to get multiple opinions before having a surgery or accepting a diagnosis. I would advise each and every person to question, question, question, and if you don't understand something, keep asking until you do. There is no ultimate authority on health and there are many ways to approach a problem. No one person has all the answers and if they say they do, you probably shouldn't trust them. Human beings are imperfect by nature, in a constant state of learning and growing. Doctors are no different.

When I rolled into the hospital for check in, at first everything proceeded as planned, as nice, compassionate nurses asked me the standard questions, I met my anesthesiologist, got hooked up on IV, etc. Then at about 1:00 p.m. someone came to tell me that Dr. Brian was running late today, about an hour or so. Well, actually make that three—I wasn't wheeled in for surgery until almost 5:00 p.m.

The surgery with Dr. Brian lasts over four hours, until well after

9:00 p.m. When I woke up in my hospital bed afterward, I remember nothing but darkness and being very scared.

"Hello," I called out, "Hello, is anyone there?"

I remember feeling so alone in that room with just the beep of the heart rate monitor. It was so quiet. Todd was there, sitting in a chair in the corner dozing off. I remember calling out more than once, or maybe I just didn't hear him answer the first time. I have never been so relieved to hear his voice say, "I'm here, honey, I'm here." He came over to the bed and held my hand.

"What have I done," I said before drifting back to sleep. I couldn't move. I felt paralyzed. I thought, I am in hell.

The next time I woke up I screamed at Todd to get a nurse. The catheter they had put in during the surgery was burning like hot fire. I yelled, "take it out, take it out!" Nurses swarmed my bedside, clearly unsure how to proceed. I was not allowed to be moved or walk. Without a catheter, how would I use the bathroom? But I was still screaming, hysterical. They really had no choice—it had to be removed. The relief was immediate. And I'm pretty sure they put something extra in my IV to sedate me because I fell back asleep shortly after. I woke up on and off throughout the night and at one point I told Todd to go home and relieve my parents. I felt strongly that Lexi should wake up with her dad there, not wanting things to be any more difficult for her. I wanted to create as much normalcy as possible during this completely abnormal time.

Now that the catheter was out, I needed assistance to pee. If I had to go, I'd buzz the nurse. Then it would take at least three nurses to help lift up my butt and slide a small tub underneath me. I had to pee right then and there with my butt perched on top of a plastic basin while three people watched, urine rolling and sliding between my legs and butt cheeks. Then when I was done the nurses had to wipe me before settling me gently back down. I remember feeling so low in these moments, so lost and so destroyed. This was by far the worst I had ever felt after a surgery and the pain was excruciating. I honestly have no idea what kind of pain meds they gave me, but they were not enough.

I don't even really remember getting discharged from the hospital or what I did there for the three days after the operation. The next part of the journey I remember is getting home and facing one of the most horrible realizations yet—Todd had brought home a rental continual passive motion (CPM) machine. The purpose of this machine was to move my hip joint without me having to exert any effort. What I would find out shortly after seeing the machine for the first time is that I would have to be hooked up to it for eight hours a day, for two weeks! In order to use the CPM machine, I would have to remain lying on my back, leg elevated on the platform while the machine moved my leg back and forth for EIGHT hours a day! Eight! That's fifty-six hours a week, a total of 112 hours attached to this machine. I was mortified—I had no idea before the surgery that this would be required for recovery. Again, I didn't ask, and if you don't ask, you can't know.

In addition to the CPM machine I had to be hooked up to an ice machine to keep my hip continuously cold. My family-room couch now officially looked like a hospital bed. I spent the better part of three weeks on that couch listening to the drone of the CPM machine, only getting up to eat and use the bathroom. I sat there in my Vicodin haze and didn't go anywhere or do anything. I just had to accept that I was stuck and time would have to pass in order for me to move forward. I was officially depressed.

About a month after this surgery I began to see Jen, my counselor, again. At one particularly difficult visit she suggested perhaps I should talk with my primary care doctor about an antidepressant. Okay, let's back up a second here because I think it's important to share what I thought about people who took antidepressants. I kind of touched on this before, but let me make it crystal clear.

I thought they were weak.

I thought they could not handle their own problems.

Dare I even say, I thought they were pathetic.

As I write this now, I'm so embarrassed. But it's the truth. I firmly believed that people who needed drugs to get through their daily lives were less than me. So, to hear Jen say that she thought I would benefit from an antidepressant was like a dagger in my heart. People like me don't need antidepressants—I am strong. I'm a business owner, an athlete. I'm powerful, I don't need any drugs. But the truth was, I really did—I was a total mess. I was having a lot of trouble getting out of bed in the morning and finding a reason to keep moving forward. I was in so much discomfort still and I couldn't see any end in sight. Honestly, if it wasn't for Lexi's bright smile and my husband's unwavering loyalty, I don't know how I would have made it at all. Everything in my life had been turned upside down. I was miserable.

Jen, my therapist:

I wasn't thinking when you came in that day that I would give you a recommendation to seek an antidepressant. I saw some of the telltale signs that perhaps medical help might be needed when you came in. You said, "it is hard to find joy, I journal but it just makes me more miserable, I am tired of my life (and lastly) I am just waiting to feel good after the pain goes away." You were not progressing, and you seemed to be continuing to decline regardless of our work. It was intuitive. I knew that I needed to do something to help move you forward.

Soon after that visit with Jen, I started a prescription for 10 milligrams of Lexipro, a Selective Serotonin Reuptake Inhibitor (SSRI). The active ingredient is Escitalopram which is used to treat depression and anxiety. It works by helping to restore the balance of serotonin in the brain. I cried so hard that day. For me, at the time, this was the ultimate defeat. I had to give in to the realization that I was not enough to hold myself together. I needed help. I needed this drug, this prescription to make through. And I tell you what, it was one of the best decisions I ever made for myself (other than maybe getting hair extensions in my late forties). Within a month of tinkering with the dosage, I settled on 15 milligrams a day. This dosage seemed to be a good place for me and I could tell a marked difference in my mood and ability to cope daily with this new fight to get my life back on track. I knew I had made the right decision and I was so grateful to Jen for nudging me in this direction. I was scared at the time that this decision would come back to haunt me someday, but the truth is, it never did. I came to realize that everyone falls on hard times and as a society, we're lucky enough to have options to help aid us in getting to a better place. I thought perhaps now that I had gone down the road of taking an antidepressant that I would need it for the rest of my life. But that was a chance I was willing to take because at that moment Lexipro provided significant gains for me. It helped me not only face my daily life with more hope, it kept me from entering the same critical low points that were fueling what sometimes felt like total darkness.

As time passed, like it always does, I started going to see a physical therapist named Zach. He was hand-picked by Dr. Brian and had worked with many of his patients. Zach was young and clearly loved his job. He was incredibly passionate about his work helping rehab people who could barely walk when they first came through his door. Zach and I worked hard together and I did get better and stronger, but the problem was, even with all this new strength, I was in pain every day. When I kept complaining that my ongoing discomfort would not go away despite months of PT, Zach did not seem to totally believe me. And I certainly felt judged by my continued use of narcotic painkillers. Zach eventually staged his own intervention.

One afternoon when I hopped up on the massage table Zach asked me a few questions about how often I was taking the painkillers. It was still a daily ritual and I told him so, admitting that every day I struggled to make it to the afternoon. That once two or three o'clock rolled around I was desperate to get some much-needed pain relief. After hearing this, Zach with his sweet, kind, twenty-something face proceeded to tell me that it was likely I was not really in pain anymore and if I stopped taking the pain killers I would realize it. He said that my brain was telling me that my hip was hurting just so I would feed it more of the opioid it enjoyed so much. I was like, whoa, buddy. You need to step off right now. You don't know anything about me or what I deal with every day. But still, hearing this hurt. It hurt because honestly, deep down, I thought maybe he was right, maybe I liked the feeling of relief in the afternoon a little too much. Maybe my hip was just fine. The images looked good, Dr. Brian had reconstructed my labrum. So why was I still in so much pain all the time?

Shortly after this conversation, Zach told me that he could not help me any further, he had done everything in his power to make me better. And even though I had improved, I struggled daily. He thought that my method of coping with the pain (taking opioids) was unhealthy and basically sent me on my way.

Our country is currently in an opioid crisis. People are dying abusing narcotic painkillers and the drug companies are under attack for making them. There are class action lawsuits against big pharma. And we are always hearing about deaths related to misuse of opioids. Now I'm not here to say everything's fine and opioids are just great for everyone, but I am here to provide another narrative. Chronic pain is a disease in and of itself. Living in pain is debilitating. It's a feeling you can't run away from, you can't escape. If you're lucky, you can find a position or two that relieves the pain. For me that was lying down—when I was lying flat on my back, I didn't feel pain. This was my go-to for relief. But, you know what, you can't live your life lying flat on your back. I had to get up and walk around, it was absolutely necessary. And I wanted to still exercise because it was good for my body and my mind. I could not do these things, especially exercise, without dulling the pain in my hip. I was still taking 15 to 20 milligrams of Vicodin a day and trying to use it as sparingly as possible. Many times, I would take three pills all at once in the afternoon after being on my feet all day. I did want to get better and I was trying, really trying, to do that. I attended physical therapy twice a week and did exercises at home. Was I crazy? Had these painkillers blinded me to the reality that I was actually fine? After a great deal of self-reflection,

I concluded that there was still something wrong and there was no way I was going to let some snot-nosed punk physical therapist tell me any different. Ultimately, I realized that I believed in myself and my narrative—I was in pain, and it was real.

I saw Dr. Brian for the last time in February 2015, seven months post operation. At our last visit I was still complaining of daily discomfort and pain when he gave me my "last" prescription for Vicodin, telling me "I'll give you this, but I don't want to create a problem here." Then he bid me farewell basically saying, "Well, I tried. There's nothing more I can do," good luck. Then he sent me on my way, still no better off—and probably worse—than when I started.

What now?

CHAPTER 12

Philly

I HAD ALREADY seen two of the hip preservation specialists in the area by now and there really weren't any more to see. I heard rumors of a doctor at Panorama Orthopedics who had studied under the impressive Dr. Mark up at the Stedman Clinic in Vail. Why not, right? Maybe he would have some new ideas.

I met Doctor Michael in early March 2015. Relatively young like the other hip preservation guys, he had a good bedside manner and listened attentively while I told him my story. Like everyone else, he seemed baffled by my condition but swore he would help me get to the bottom of it. Since I had just filled a prescription from Dr. Brian, I didn't have to talk with Dr. Michael about pain management, and he never asked. These days, doctors don't want to prescribe pain medication for anything—no matter how miserable you are. If you want help with managing pain, you're definitely going to have to ask. Then the doctors will make you feel really uncomfortable before they suggest Advil or simply tell you they don't prescribe opioids, period. I believe that was Dr. Michael's policy, even though he never actually said it out loud.

The first order of business would be a series of ultrasound injections based on where my pain seemed to be coming from. I would point and they would poke. Okay, that's simplifying it a little bit, but it's pretty accurate. I scheduled two sets of these injections, the first did nothing to help. But the second was a bit more promising. It suggested a very unique diagnosis, especially for a woman—athletic pubulgia. This condition, also called a sports hernia, hockey hernia, hockey groin, Gilmore's groin, or groin disruption is a medical condition of the pubic joint that affects athletes. Much of my pain was centered in the groin area, so this very rare issue was a possible cause. According to OthroInfo.org, more than 90% of patients who go through nonsurgical treatment (PT, rest, Advil, etc.) and then surgery are able to return to sports activity. Ninety percent! Now those odds sounded really good to me. Once again, we didn't REALLY know if this core muscle tear at the pubic joint was the cause of my ongoing battle, but it seemed like the most promising lead we had to date.

But this time, I was going to do a way better job of picking my surgeon—I was determined to find the best, most capable individual in the entire country to help me. No more pussy footing around. I would go wherever I needed to go to do this right!

After extensive research I landed on Dr. William of the Vincera Clinic in Philadelphia, Pennsylvania. He was "the guy." His work was cutting edge, and he had operated on some very famous athletes, including fellow Coloradan and Rockies player Tory Tulowitski. Even the website boasts "professional, college and amateur athletes, as well as people suffering from undiagnosed pain, travel from across the world to Vincera for treatment." But before I went across the country and paid "out of pocket" for this surgery I was going to make sure I had every document relating to my hip sent to the clinic. I wanted to make sure they saw all the supporting evidence before they cut me open, so they would know it was the right thing to do. I had seen several other doctors not mentioned in this book and I made sure every one of them sent a medical record to Vincera. Dr. Michael, my main doctor at the time, supported the visit although I'm not sure he was really convinced this was the right diagnosis. But he didn't have any other ideas either, so off I went.

I scheduled the surgery for April 2015. I would be in Philadelphia for about a week and my dad would accompany me on the trip. The surgery was outpatient and I was told I would be able to walk right after. My dad and I booked a hotel and rental car and headed out on another surgical adventure together.

My dad had been my sidekick through most of the surgeries thus far. Because Todd and my mom were tag-teaming Lexi, my dad was usually stuck dealing with me. True to form, he never complained and was always very loyal. We used to joke that when I stopped having surgeries we might not get a chance to talk as much. Kind of funny, but not really. So, I wasn't surprised when he stepped up and said he would go with me to Philly.

The surgery center was located in the historic Philadelphia Navy Yard. It was stunning and the spring weather was beautiful. My dad and I got to enjoy walks along the pier gazing at the giant boats that made us feel like dwarfs. It was surreal that we had flown all the way from Colorado and I was about to pay around $20,000 to have yet another surgery. The Vincera Institute bills itself as an upscale alternative to a traditional hospital, and I must say it was impressive. The building housed the physician's clinic, specific diagnostic imaging, out-patient surgery, physical therapy, yoga, massage, acupuncture, nutrition and even counseling if you needed it.

I met with Dr. William the day after our arrival. I was assuming he had reviewed all of my records and knew exactly how he would handle my case. Ha! Wrong. As I should have come to expect by now, of course, I would need another MRI, and this one would be better than any other one I had ever had (insert eye roll here). If you look up diagnostic imaging on the Vincera website this is what it says: Dr. William "and leading radiologists at Thomas Jefferson University in Philadelphia were the first group to develop MR imaging techniques and protocols dedicated to the diagnosis of core and pelvis injuries. This MRI technique is 92% accurate and can reveal other problems, such as "soft" musculoskeletal findings, tiny avulsions fractures, peculiar edema patterns, or intrinsic hip pathology. It is both sensitive and specific for various injuries about the pubic symphysis specifically for rectus abdominis and adductor pathology and also involving the hip and visceral pelvis. Additionally, this MRI of the pelvis uses both surface coil and send-receive body coil, as well as oblique planes to maximize sensitivity and specificity for osseous and musculotendinous pathology of the pelvis." I didn't know what half of that meant, so how could I even argue. If another MRI would help the doctors make a better decision for me, then by all means, let's get it done.

The great thing about Vincera is it's an incredibly streamlined program. Once you get there, they take you from start to finish fairly quickly. It's not like visiting your local doctor, getting a referral, going to an imaging service, going back to the doctor, pre-op appointments, etc. They get all this done in one day at Vincera. And if you're a candidate for Dr. William's fine surgical work, they schedule the operation for the following day.

After my MRI was complete, I was called into the office to review the findings with Dr. William, my dad, and we even FaceTimed Todd so everyone could hear what the doctor was going to say. It was disappointing, to say the least. Dr. William said that indeed I had a small core muscle tear, but he was not sure if the surgery would really do anything to help my chronic pain. He said we could go through with it, in hopes that it would make a difference, but he was really unsure that the results would give me the relief I was looking for. He said he had consulted with a colleague in Vail (Dr. Mark from Stedman again) about my case and suggested if this surgery did not help, that I go see him in the upcoming months. Dr. William mentioned that I had minor hip dysplasia and suggested that it might be the underlying source of the pain. But he just wasn't sure.

UGH!!! What do I do? I mean I had flown all the way there, I had such high hopes for pain relief. He said, the surgery might help. Was "might" a good enough chance to go through yet another surgery? We (me, my dad and Todd) all agreed that yes, "might" was good enough. Surgery was scheduled for the next day.

I checked into the clinic the next morning and my dad made a comfortable spot for himself in the waiting room, both of us expecting me to be on the operating table for hours. But surprisingly the core muscle repair only took about thirty minutes from start to finish. When I woke up the first thing I noticed was they had shaved all my pubic hair! Hey, man, what the heck, no one told me they were going to do that! The incision for the repair was right on my pubic bone and it was only about an inch long. I waited in recovery until I was coherent enough to leave the surgery center and head back to my hotel with my dad. The bonus of this procedure was that I could walk right after, there were no ill effects from movement. Our hotel was close by and comfortable. Once I settled into my bed with my fresh new Percocet (10 milligrams oxycodone and 325 milligrams of acetaminophen) prescription, off to sleep I went.

For the next five days, my dad would drive me to the clinic where I would get post-surgical physical therapy from core muscle repair specialists. While I was there, I would see more than one college athlete with their coach going through the same protocol, and even a professional basketball player. In fact, I was one of the few patients who didn't have a sports team name on his chest. And I say his, because I was the only female there at the time. I had two therapists, Nicole during the week, and on the weekend the PT for the Philadelphia Flyers professional hockey team (his name escapes me now). They were both exceptionally kind and helpful. Of course, while I was there I was still in pain, but I had also just had surgery. I was told that within a couple of weeks I should be just fine, IF the surgery had worked and the core muscle injury was the true source of my ongoing battle.

Well surprise, surprise—it wasn't.

I was as miserable as ever when I returned to Colorado. I did all of my physical therapy religiously, working to get better every day. But it was just not working—the pain was the same and it was all encompassing. It was the first thing I thought of when I woke up in the morning and the last thing in my mind as a drifted off to sleep. I was miserable and so unsure of what the future would hold for me. I was heartbroken, lost and no amount of antidepressants seemed to help. Seven surgeries in seven years. I was broken on the inside and the outside and desperate for answers.

CHAPTER 13

AhhhhhxyContin

IN MAY 2015 I visited my primary care doctor for a refill of my antidepressant. She knew the story of what I had been through over the last
several years and she felt horrible for me. I told her about the pain I
felt every day and the discomfort I dealt with each and every minute.
I told her that the only relief I got was lying in bed at night and even
then, the residual effects of a day of moving my hip lingered, making
sleep fleeting and difficult. She asked me what I was taking for the
pain and I told her about the Vicodin and Percocet. I told her nothing
over-the-counter worked and that I was just dealing with it. I was going to therapy, seeing doctor after doctor, taking antidepressants and I
told her I was not giving up. I assured her I would not rest until I found
out what was wrong with me, if it was the last thing I ever did. And
that is when she asked if I had ever heard of OxyContin.

I remember telling her no, even though I had, of course, heard
of it. I didn't want her to think I knew about the drug for fear that it
would skew her judgement about whether or not to give it to me. The
truth was, I had never taken Oxy (except briefly post-surgery), even
in my drug taking days. Painkillers were not really part of the scene
when I was experimenting in college. I really had no idea about the
drug's addictive properties or about the growing case society was
building against Purdue Pharma, the manufacturer of OxyContin.
The only thing I really knew for sure was that it was stronger than the

Vicodin I was taking every day. My doctor was very concerned about the amount of acetaminophen I was putting in my system and she thought perhaps I would benefit from the extended relief properties of Oxy. The concept behind this drug is you can take one 10 milligram dosage (the minimum dose in pill form) and it would give pain relief for up to twelve hours. TWELVE hours! I couldn't imagine such bliss. I couldn't imagine complete pain relief period, much less for an extended period of time. It sounded too good to be true.

When I recently asked this doctor, who I still see to this day, if she ever worried about giving me my first prescription of Oxy, if she ever thought I would become addicted or turn into some junkie, she answered a resounding "No, I was not worried, not at all. I knew you were in pain and I knew you were not going to give up until you found the source. I trusted my gut. I have only prescribed Oxy twice in my medical career; that was true the day I gave you your first prescription and it is still true today." My doctor is a family practice doctor, not a surgeon or a pain specialist. And when I reflect on her decision to prescribe me this drug—I sometimes wonder what would have happened if she hadn't.

Jen Sutton, my therapist:

I remember when you told me you had started taking extended relief opioids. I was totally concerned. We had talked on multiple occasions about how you were concerned about taking Vicodin because it not only helped with the pain but it helped mask your negative thoughts. And this was a big step up. I knew you needed something for pain...but I thought, she's going to like this and that isn't going to be good. I was very worried. I couldn't say, Erin, you can't take that, but I thought we might end up with a serious addiction down the road.

I picked up that first prescription at the Target pharmacy close to my house under the scrutinizing eye of the lead pharmacist who had already filled countless fast-acting opioid prescriptions for me.

I was certain she was judging me just like Zach, the PT, had done. Whatever. I just wanted to wash that pill down my throat and feel the promised sweet relief. I don't think I even made it to the parking lot before I had swallowed that first dose. And I waited and waited. Did it help? Yea, a little, but nothing like what I wanted. I wanted to feel nothing, no pain. I wanted to pretend I was fine and my hip did not hurt. I wanted to run and play with my daughter. I wanted to be happy. I wanted to be free.

I learned a lot about my tolerance for opioids during that first month on Oxy. I learned that the dose only worked for about eight hours—I didn't get anything close to the twelve hours of relief my doctor had suggested. But eight was better than nothing and I still had Vicodin for those extra bad times. In order to fill the whole day with some sort of pain relief, my doctor eventually prescribed 10 milligrams three times a day, every eight hours. And after about a month of this, I moved up to 20 milligrams twice a day and 10 milligrams to sleep at night. So, by July 2015 I was taking about 50 to 60 milligrams of Oxy a day and it was working! Even though I still spent a large amount of time meeting doctors and investigating next steps, I was not in "that much" pain anymore. I was able to get back to exercise and even to running. Was that a good idea? No, of course it wasn't. But I was happy. I could move, I could go to the park with my daughter and could even have sex! It was so amazing.

To be perfectly honest I never considered the potential repercussions of taking this drug. I mean I knew it was serious, but I didn't care—I just didn't want to hurt anymore. Living in pain all the time, every day, was like being suffocated with a pillow. I couldn't breathe. I couldn't function. All I could do was focus on my misery, and I would have done absolutely anything to escape it. I didn't do research about Oxy or ask tough questions. I just took it, day in and day out. It was wonderful.

And why should I have worried at all? According to the American Society of Anesthesiologists I could "avoid (the) side effects and risk of addiction, (if I) used them only under a physician's supervision.

Physician anesthesiologists and medical doctors who specialize in anesthesia, pain management and critical care medicine — have extensive training and experience in prescribing opioid and non-opioid pain medications...(they can) make sure (my) pain is under control while minimizing side effects and the risk of addiction." Well that was exactly what I was doing. So, I felt like generally I was safe from whatever horrible things might happen to people taking OxyContin. And ultimately safe from addiction.

In order to keep the prescription coming I had to see my doctor every month. She would check in with me and see where I was with my quest for answers. She would ask me questions about my life and probably generally just "check" on me. I always scheduled my appointment several days before my prescription would run out. This way I could take an extra dose for a particularly long run or if I had to sit in the car for several hours—two things that really aggravated my hip. The pharmacist would fill the prescription up to four days early. And I always filled four days early! That was 200 milligrams extra I got to play around with, based on my needs. I wanted this flexibility in order to maximize my pain relief and my ability to try and live a "normalish" life.

But make no mistake—just because I had found a temporary solution for my pain did not mean I became complacent about figuring out why, exactly, my hip was still hurting so badly. I found a new PT, Dr. Eric, who specialized in more non-traditional forms of pain relief like the Graston Technique, dry needling and chiropractic adjustments. I had really done everything I could to get stronger in the traditional physical therapy way. Dr. Eric had a new approach to helping me while I considered other medical options. According to grastontechique.com, the Graston Technique® is defined as "a unique, evidence-based form of instrument-assisted soft tissue mobilization that enables clinicians to effectively and efficiently address soft tissue lesions and fascial restrictions resulting in improved patient outcomes." So basically, Dr. Eric would "scrape" the muscles around my hip joint trying to release some of the tension there. He also would place tiny needles into my muscles with the same end goal, getting them to release. All the while, he would chit chat with me about life. I learned all about who he was dating and why he wasn't married yet. I learned about his background working with Olympians and why he had left that scene. I told him about my struggles with pain and my hip. He was a good listener and became a friend as well as a practitioner.

Once I was absolutely positive that the surgery in Philly had been unsuccessful I made a series of appointments with several new doctors. I went back to Dr. Michael and he recommended another round of diagnostic injections which proved ineffective once again.

Finally, he suggested a full hip replacement. At just forty-two years old, a hip replacement would be life-changing. Not only would my ability to run be limited, to say the least, I would be faced with future hip replacements as well. An active person can expect a replacement to last ten, maybe fifteen years, which means I would need a few more of them before I keeled over for good. Each one would likely result in more challenges and less mobility. This was a BIG deal and a decision I was not quite ready to make. I mean I still wanted to run, and at the time I WAS running, thanks to OxyContin. So, I thought maybe I should go back to where I started and see Dr. Omer again. Even though I was still pissed about the outcome of the original hip surgery I felt I had nowhere left to turn. I thought maybe he could offer some insight as to what I should do next because honestly, I had no idea.

I scheduled a visit at his new office which had now been upgraded from the dingy clinic on Maplewood to a state-of-the-art facility located on the University of Colorado campus. It was beautiful, shiny and new with bright white walls and an enormous waiting area with inspiring Olympic moments playing on a TV and signed posters from amazing collegiate and professional athletes. The minute you walked in, it felt like you were in the right place, where dreams are revived and the phoenix can rise from the ashes. For just a moment I felt like maybe I could be one of those people.

After touching base and reviewing what I been through since our last meeting, Dr. Omer took X-rays and reviewed my most recent MRI and we discussed options. He echoed Dr. Michael's recommendation that perhaps a hip replacement was the answer. He offered to help coordinate my care through this process, but I was still wary of him and CU at the time, so I bid him farewell and continued on my quest.

Next I made an appointment with the famous Dr. Mark from the Stedman Clinic in Vail. He was the undisputed leader in the field of hip preservation, so I believed that maybe he would be able to find something the other doctors could not. Maybe he, in his infinite wisdom, would have a path for me that did not require a full hip replacement.

The appointment was in Vail on a beautiful dazzling summer day. I arrived early in the morning and the front desk told me I better get comfortable because I would be there all day. As expected, Stedman also had super-special MRI machines, so in order for me to see one of their doctors I had to get yet another set of images done. They also made me see a physical therapist who took a number of measurements of my hip. He bent my leg this way and that, measuring mobility and asking me if it hurt, etc. Then after all of that crap, I waited—and waited, and waited for Dr. Mark to get out of surgery so he could see me. I got to the Vail clinic around 8:00 a.m. and didn't see him until 6:00 p.m. Couple that amount of time with the anxiety of waiting to talk to someone that might potentially have an answer for you, ugh—it was an awful day.

When I finally entered Dr. Mark's office in the evening, it wasn't at all what I had expected. He didn't see me in an exam room, instead I just went into his giant office where my images had been pulled up on a video screen. His desk was messy, strewn with papers and books. His assistant stood by dutifully waiting for Dr. Mark's thoughts on my case. I gave him the brief lowdown on what I had been through thus far and he said how sorry he was, and how he could not imagine what it was like to be me. I immediately liked him. His face was kind, and even though I was so pissed about waiting all frickin' day for him, his manner put me at ease. He proceeded to tell me pretty much exactly what Dr. Omer and Dr. Michael had said—it was time to get a hip replacement. Ultimately, he basically told me he couldn't help. When the very best, most well-known hip preservation surgeon in arguably the world says he can't help—there really is nothing more you can do.

I went to my car and I cried.

You would think crying would be a part of my everyday life. I mean, I was in pain all the time and spent at least half of my free time meeting with doctors. I was completely miserable in every sense of the word working an unrewarding job and living in a desperate state of limbo. But you know what, that is one of Oxy's many beautiful qualities—I was just numb. I was going through the motions, trying to get answers and living the best life I could. But mostly, I couldn't really feel anything deep enough to hurt me. I would just swallow another pill and continue to move through life. When I reflect on this, I'm so incredibly grateful for this side effect of the drug, because it kept me moving forward. It kept me searching. It made life livable. I know that sounds awful and kind of disgusting, but it's true. When I cried that evening in the Stedman Clinic parking lot, it was one of the first times I had cried in months, and it was violent. My tears were rivers down my cheeks soaking my T-shirt. My head hung so low, almost touching my sternum, and my body racked with sobs. The hope for answers had been squelched, and on that day I knew I had no choice. My days as a runner were over—it was time to commit to the hip replacement.

CHAPTER 14

Bionic

I WAS SO sad that my time as a runner was going to be over not just for a season, but for a lifetime. Sure, I would be able to waddle around in the woods, but twelve-mile jaunts in the foothills would be a thing of the past. Since I was still predominantly seeing Dr. Michael, he recommended a surgeon, Dr. Peter, to do the replacement. I met with him in September 2015. He seemed nice, soft spoken and confident the replacement would indeed get rid of my pain for good. And honestly, at this point, that was all I wanted. I mean, ALL I WANTED! Even though it still breaks my heart that I can't run, at the time, I barely cared at all, and felt like I had no way out except the replacement. I mean I had tried virtually everything and was now taking 60 or 70 milligrams of Oxy a day in order to keep myself functioning at a high enough level to pretend like my life was not a total mess.

Life on drugs was now the only life I knew. And the scariest thing about it was to most people I seemed totally fine—I drove carpools, volunteered at school, worked and interacted with my family. And doing all of this on OxyContin 24/7 seemed completely normal. I was taking enough of the drug to essentially operate like I wasn't in all that much pain. As long as I took them every day I was just fine. But the most disturbing part of my new-found dependency was how often I counted my pills. Since I always filled my prescription a few days early—I always had a few extra days of pills to work with. So,

I could take more than my allotted amount. I usually did this so I could exercise harder, run longer or attend a trade show or some other event where I had to stand for long periods of time. But those days happened all the time and I always wanted more pills. I counted them religiously. I'm not sure if I was hoping more would magically appear or if I was just nuts. I also had prescriptions for muscle relaxers, Valium and Tramadol. Sometimes I would add a little of this or a little of that to help get me through my day. To most people, I still think I seemed pretty normal.

But, oh, I was far from it.

Surgery was scheduled for October 27, 2015 and would mark my eighth surgery since 2009. The surgery would take place at a hospital who's name I literally can't recall, I mean I could look it up, but why. That is how messed up I was, I don't even know where the surgery happened. It looked to be as routine as any replacement surgery. According to the Orthopedic Design and Technology website there were 370,700 total hip replacements performed in 2014, and that number grows every year. I had every reason to believe that even though I would never be that sexy runner again, I would finally be pain-free and this nightmare would be over for good. I had high expectations for the outcome and was generally really excited for it all to be over.

I planned a final run with my girlfriend, Keira, for October 26. Keira has been in my life since the early 2000's. She's one of my people, and even though we have almost no mutual friends, we still make time to see each other. I call Keira my exercise buddy. She and I share similar passions and enjoyed not just catching up over coffee, but catching up over activities. We went for runs together and climbed at the gym quite a bit. One of us was always slightly better than the other on any given day, so we provided good motivation and support. We discussed training and racing, kids (Keira has a son), our husbands, work, everything. She was the perfect person to share this last nugget of running love. We headed up the South Boulder Creek trail on an unseasonably snowy day. I could always count on Keira to show up no matter what the weather was doing, and knew this day would be no different. We both loved being out there when no one else was—getting one more run under our belts while the rest of the world was snuggling in their PJ's by the fire.

With wet snow sloshing under our shoes and mud making our footing tumultuous, we powered up into the Boulder foothills. Snowflakes stung our faces as we grinned from ear to ear. We were in love with the moment, the quiet and the purity of it all. I gave thanks to the universe for all of the miles I had traveled on my legs; for all of the gymnastics competitions and the dance performances I had enjoyed throughout my life. I had lived so "hard" thus far and with so much passion, giving everything I had to every pursuit. I worked myself to the bone to be strong and to fight. I vowed on that day to never stop living, and even though I would not run like this again, I knew I would still do great things. I would not let this hip replacement change me or diminish the fire that had always been burning inside me. On that day I made peace with what lay ahead. On that day I was ready for my new future.

Keira:

I remember our final run together very clearly. It was incredible out with a few inches of fresh snow on the ground and more falling from the skies. The kind of day where you see hardly anyone and feel like a superhero just getting out the door. It felt so natural to be lacing up my shoes to head out with Erin. I did feel a little conflicted emotionally. On the one hand, I was honored that she chose me as her partner for that day but I also remember thinking that this wasn't our final run, we were just kicking off a large break while she took time to work through injuries. She was a fighter and if there was a will, she would find the way. Ignorance or wishful thinking, I'm not sure, but I was positive that she would run again even though she was telling me that she wouldn't.

In hindsight, I think I probably didn't show up for her in the way that she needed. Maybe knowing that unconsciously, I had a sense of nervous anticipation as we headed out from the trailhead. I felt a little pressure, from myself, to make this run amazing for her. The terrain was slippery and rocky underfoot and we took care to mind our feet to avoid any injurious falls. As my mind settled into the activity, my worries faded and I simply enjoyed the time with her. The run felt magical with the snow but the magic was in the synchronous breathing of two friends working their bodies and minds.

Before I knew it, we were back to the trailhead soaked from sweat and snow. We didn't linger long as we knew our body temperatures would drop as quickly as our heart rates. As I drove away, I felt gratitude for another amazing run with my friend. I don't recall her experiences having any effects on my vision of myself as an athlete. I'm not sure if I didn't have enough experience with injury yet or just felt like with modern medicine there would always be a fix. I looked forward to helping her recover and begin the slow rebuilding process. Even if she never got back to 100%, I knew she'd work hard and get closer than anyone was telling her was possible.

Believe it or not, I honestly don't remember much about the hip replacement surgery either, probably because I was on so, so many drugs at the time. But I sure do remember what happened after, clear as day. Once I got out of the hospital I stayed at my parent's house for about a week, as I needed constant care and help. Todd was traveling some and I needed the support of the people who love me most in this world—my family. I was so grateful not just to have a place to stay but to have the company of my parents throughout the day. They were nothing short of amazing. They never complained and never made me feel like a burden. They were 100 percent all in and taking care of me was their primary goal. When Todd was gone Lexi and I both stayed at their house.

In early November, less than a week out from surgery, my mom had prepared dinner for me, Lexi and my dad. She always made my favorite dishes when I was staying with her and tonight was no different. It was shrimp pasta primavera. I could smell it from my spot on the couch where I spent the majority of my day. But when I went to stand up, grab my walker and come to the dinner table, something terrible happened.

There are some moments in life that grab hold of you and never let go. Sometimes those moments are glorious and sometimes they are traumatic. On that November evening, I would experience what would ultimately lead to the height of my nightmare. This moment, this simple movement to stand would send me into a tailspin of panic. As I stood up on my newly replaced hip, it just collapsed. I felt it pop out of place sending shooting pain from the top of my head to the tip of my toes. I screamed to my parents to call 911 while my daughter sat there in horror watching her mom writhing once again on the ground. It was the most painful thing I have ever felt. And in a life full of constant pain, that is a bold statement. It lasted for maybe two or three minutes and then pop, it went right back in and the pain stopped.

When the ambulance arrived, I was no longer screaming and I had caught my breath. I was in shock. I had just experienced something horrible and I had no idea what had happened or what it meant for my new hip. The paramedics thought it best to take me to the hospital and have things checked out. I wanted Lexi to stay with my parents, so I called my friend Jen to come be with me at the hospital. I was so beside myself with fear I could barely even talk. The ER doctor suggested I get a CT scan of the area to make sure nothing had happened to the replacement. Nothing happened? *Really?* Something had definitely fucking happened. I just collapsed on the living room floor and called 911. How could this ever be just "one of those things?" Something was wrong—I was sure of it.

I was always honest with the hospitals and doctors about my painkiller regiment and post-surgery I was taking about 80 to 100 milligrams of Oxy a day along with lots of other drugs too. Maybe the

ER doc just thought I was crazy or a junkie or whatever. It was clear no one really believed me. I mean, one minute I was calling 911 and the next I was fine—sounded suspicious, I guess.

Jen, my best friend:

There was never a time in this entire journey that I did not believe Erin. She has never been an exaggerator. She doesn't blow the truth out of proportion. For Erin, a six-inch fish is never a 16-inch fish. So, I knew in the hospital that day, like every other day, that this was real.

Erin is not an attention seeker. It is not her personality. When I asked my husband if he remembered me questioning Erin's situation, he said, "you questioned her decisions, but never her reality." I have always believed every word that came out of her mouth. This time was no different.

But when I left the hospital that day, I was scared. Her fears were my fears. Calling 911 doesn't just "happen"—especially not with Erin.

The orthopedist on call reviewed my CT scan and told me everything looked just fine. They didn't really know what happened, but according to the images, I seemed to be okay. I wanted to believe this very badly, so I did. I was relieved and grateful that even though this incredibly strange thing had happened, I was no worse for wear and everything would be just fine. And for a while that seemed to be the case. I went to all of my post-op appointments and all of the imaging seemed normal, but I was still in pain long after it should have subsided. Everyone—doctors, physical therapists, etc.—believed I only needed time to get better. I needed to be patient and rest, to pace myself and take things on slowly.

But most of all, to understand the true nature of whatever pain still remained, I needed to stop taking the painkillers.

CHAPTER 15

Dopesick

BEFORE MY HIP replacement, my primary care doctor had referred me to a pain specialist, Dr. Lief. His office was located right above hers, so communication between them was easy. She felt like my OxyContin prescription needs were getting to be too much for her to handle—meaning I constantly needed/wanted more. She felt like it was beyond her scope of work, which it certainly was.

Since Dr. Lief met me pretty far into my pain journey, he kind of just had to go with what I had been doing thus far and support the meds I was currently taking. He took over my case right before the replacement, so basically, he would just maintain my narcotic needs until it was time to get off the drugs.

I knew after getting the hip replacement I would need to stop taking the painkillers. How could I really assess my healing if I was continuing to mask the pain with drugs? And I was taking so many drugs—I had a Tupperware full of prescription pill bottles next to the couch where I spent most of my time. I had Valium, Percocet, OxyContin in several dosages, muscle relaxers, anti-nausea medicine, blood thinners, antidepressants and probably a few others I can't even remember. Some were easier to stop taking than others of course. The blood thinners and anti-nausea meds were the first to go. I never felt that the Valium or muscle relaxers were all that effective, so it was also easy to put those in the medicine cabinet for a rainy day. I planned to continue with the antidepressants for the foresee-able future, but the painkillers, ahh those trusty painkillers…when the pain was gone or bearable, I would need to stop taking the opioids, and that terrified me. As I continued to improve with time and my trusty physical therapy, I started to research what it would be like to be dopesick.

I mean, I knew generally that it would suck, and I would feel awful. I knew from experience when I was pushing the time limit be-tween pills, I would start to freak out. And it wasn't just because the pain would return or be unbearable. I knew by that point I needed the Oxy like I needed air to breathe. I relished in each and every dose, knowing it would not only take away the chronic pain I faced daily, but it would also make it possible for me to cope with my reality. With Oxy I could go on with my life as if nothing was really wrong. I could mask the pain I felt both physically and emotionally. I loved those painkillers. I loved how they made me feel and I was scared to face my life without them. But it was going to happen and I needed to get ready.

First, I turned to the world wide web, probably the worst place to look for medical advice. I trolled various Oxy blogs reading about different people's experiences with withdrawal. I bought supplements they recommended including Phentolamine, Kava Kava and a few other herbs. Dr. Lief and I planned to wean myself off the drugs slow-ly by reducing my dosage by 10 milligrams a week. This all sounded so good and smart, but anyone who has been dependent on opioids will tell you this is not that easy. Oxy holds you like a vice and if you aren't giving your body at least what it's used to, you're going to suffer, and that goes against every fiber of your being. When I was supposed to reduce my intake by those 10 milligrams a week, I didn't. I took as much as I had been taking until there were just enough pills for me to reduce my intake by 10 milligrams a DAY before I had no more drugs. I knew at this point I had no choice. I had to bear down and just do it.

Being opioid dependent isn't something you talk to anyone about—not your parents, not your spouse, not your friends—no one.

Even though the people closest to you know you're taking a bunch of drugs, no one talks about it. You keep it all inside and face your dependency all alone. I didn't like that feeling so I decide to seek out people I knew would understand, those at Narcotics Anonymous.

I attended my first NA meeting at Centennial Hospital in Louisville. One thing I didn't understand before showing up was that Centennial was a drug treatment facility and several people in attendance would be those forced to be there because of their admittance to the hospital. The people I met in that meeting had gone over the edge and shared stories about stealing, shooting up, isolating everyone in their lives and living on the streets. Hearing these stories made me wonder, how is this possible? How can a drug have that kind of hold on someone? Could that someone be me? When I attended the first meeting I was still taking the drugs (even though that is an NA no-no), but I kept that to myself. I shared my story of the surgeries and the need for painkillers to control my chronic pain. I shared my fear for the future and uncertainty about life without narcotics and what that would look like...I just didn't know. Were these my people? Was I like them? Were they like me? I honestly wasn't sure, and that was so incredibly, unbearably scary.

The day finally came when I had no choice but to stop taking Oxy—I had no more left. I went from taking 80 milligrams a day to none in eight days.

Would I find myself looking for heroin or ordering pills from Mexico? Would I throw up? Would I see cockroaches crawling on my skin? I didn't know. The only thing I was sure of at that point was I was about to be miserable—very, very miserable.

I dissolved my last Oxy at my therapist's office. I told her it was time to be done with Oxy and she said, okay, hand it over. I placed my last white circular pill in her hand as the nausea and fear rose in my belly. She went to the water cooler to fill up a Dixie cup with liquid and promptly dropped the pill in water. I watched it dissolve into thousands of tiny particles. And I thought, this is it. Here goes...

For me, it was the headaches. Oh my God, the headaches. It

started almost immediately with the drop-in dosage. My head felt like it was going to explode, as if it were being squeezed between two pieces of metal. The pressure was unbearable and nothing helped. Tylenol and Advil were almost comical aids and did virtually nothing to stop the pain. I just had to sit with it, own it and accept it. This was not easy and I could often feel myself teetering on the edge of what felt like insanity. Like I wanted to quite literally jump out of my bedroom window, like I wanted to run through the streets of my suburban small town screaming and throwing things, like I wanted to stick my head in a toilet and drown. It seemed as if the pain would never end, and yet I could not share with anyone that withdrawal was "that hard." What was I supposed to tell my seven-year-old daughter? "Oh honey, Mommy is dopesick, don't worry, everything is going to be fine." Detoxing isn't something you move through in twenty-four or forty-eight hours, it takes weeks to feel human again.

It was a Friday. I thought it would be best to have the first two days fall on a weekend when I could get the most support from Todd and my family. In retrospect, I don't think there is a good day to stop taking Oxy. It could have been fucking Christmas and I would have been immersed in my own personal hell. I remember trying so hard to act normal, be normal. "How are you feeling?" my friends would ask... "Not that bad," I would answer. I mean, what was I supposed to say? "I haven't slept in a week and I'm petrified I'm going to turn into some kind of junkie in the next twenty-four hours?" Not sure that would have gone over so well with the parents of my daughter's friends. So, I smiled and gave the thumbs up, all the while trying to quell the nausea and headaches that I felt would consume me. I pretended to be okay, to be normal, when inside I was dying.

The misery of going without Oxy was extreme. As a mom and a wife, I didn't want to let on that I felt as if I were literally coming apart at the seams. I could not sleep. I don't think I slept for about nine days. I couldn't get comfortable no matter how much I tried to relax. It was as if my body and mind weren't connected—I could focus on relaxing in my mind, but my body had a different idea. They term it "restless leg syndrome" on one of the Oxy withdrawal websites. My body just couldn't stop moving. I tossed and turned and spent most of my nights in an awake/dream state just plain suffering. I listened to books like "Dreamland" and "All Fall Down." These are books about Oxy, both fiction and non-fiction. I was obsessed with my situation and I desperately wanted to understand where I was going and what was happening to me.

I barely even remember going to work or volunteering at Lexi's school. I was sweating and nauseous all the time. I told Lexi I had the flu for a couple of days and just didn't get out of bed. I just lay there on my covers desperate for sleep, slipping in and out of consciousness. But during all of this suffering, I never once thought about trying to get more of the drug. I didn't want anything to do with what had brought me to the lowest point I had ever been. I felt like I was being buried alive.

I could not for the life of me understand how after all this suffering how anyone could want to take more of this poison. I still wonder to this day, why I was spared the need that those I met at Narcotics Anonymous felt. I did not want more drugs, I wanted nothing to do with them ever again. Maybe it's my DNA, or my iron will. Maybe I'll never know. But I am so grateful I did not feel the need to squash the dopesick. I knew I just had to be in it. I had to survive it. I knew for a fact I was not going to die. I was going to live, for my beautiful daughter and my strong husband. I knew I would beat it and I would prevail. There was absolutely no doubt in my mind.

Once the fog lifted and I began to believe that I would function once again like a normal human being, I swore I would never take another opioid again. I would never let a drug take over my life again, no matter what.

Or so I thought.

PART THREE
THE PIT

CHAPTER 16

Gratitude and Grit

PEOPLE ASK ME all the time, "How did you get through all of that?" Meaning how did I survive the last ten years. This story is going to get way worse before it gets better, so at this point I want to share the two things that helped me get through most days.

Gratitude

It was not until the problems with my hip started to spiral out of control that I found the essential quality of adding the practice of gratitude to my life. As a young person, and honestly, well into my adult life, I have never been grateful. I just expected things to work out for me. I believed that if I put my heart into something and worked hard to achieve an outcome, then that would guarantee success. I didn't need to be grateful, because I had indeed controlled and orchestrated everything that had ever happened to me. I did not owe gratitude to the universe or to God because I was the one forging my own destiny.

But what happened when these facts no longer held true? I mean, I was passionate and working diligently to get better. I was following all of the protocols and seeking out the best physicians to help me. But I was getting worse. It was counterintuitive to everything I had ever known to be true. At this point in my life, I began to practice what I now term "radical acceptance" of my situation. And in order to live in that place I had to find gratitude.

Radical acceptance is the ability to be in your own moment. And in order to be in the moment, you must first accept where you are. Now, I usually don't buy into all of the woo-woo Boulder metaphysical bullshit, but by this time in my journey I had to find something to hold on to. I'm not religious, but I do consider myself a spiritual person. I believe in a higher power and the connectivity of the universe. And because of this fundamental belief, I had to conclude that this life, this path I was on, was truly mine to walk. I had to accept it for what it was—a dark, desperate time full of pain and torture and what seemed like a never-ending plummet into what I termed "The Pit," an imaginary hole in the ground where I lived, a place of complete despair and darkness. And often I felt like The Pit kept sinking deeper. I would try and make handholds and footholds to climb out, but every time I did, rain would come and wash all of my hard work away. Sometimes I felt like people were throwing dirt on me. It would get in my mouth and my eyes, making it harder for me to breathe and see. It was a form of hell and this was the place I inhabited. I had to accept that. I had to be in The Pit and learn how to exist there. There were certainly days in the latter part of this story where I admit I would rather have died than live in pain forever. But in order to keep this feeling from taking over my entire self, I had to find gratitude.

Gratitude is defined as the quality of being thankful. What could I have possibly had to be thankful for all those years in and out of doctor's offices in chronic pain, on drugs and suffering with literally every step? I will tell you what—just about everything.

I found the ability to be grateful for the smallest things—my daughter's smile, a sunset, a scenic drive, my coloring book. I absolutely had to find joy in The Pit. I had to find bits of light and hope. I had to see the beauty in my journey and believe that someday I would understand it. I am no longer in pain and I still appreciate all of those little things every day. And I'm not sure I would see the world in this way if I had not suffered so deeply for so many years. Today, I still try and live as much in the moment as I can. I try not to worry about the future or what I cannot change. I accept where I am at any given time and in doing that I find brilliant, shiny rays of joy and gratitude everywhere. Am I perfect at this practice? Hell no. No one is ever perfect at anything. Sometimes I worry about my daughter's American Ninja Warrior competitions, sometimes I get caught in stupid work dramas or look at myself in the mirror and wish I looked younger. But you know what, I have grown leaps and bounds in my practice of both acceptance and gratitude. I can catch myself now thinking toxic thoughts and check myself. I can reflect back on what I have been through and think...baaaaaaa...these little petty things (work drama, competitions, aging), they really do not matter. I think, "I am going to be here *now* and find the beauty in *this* place." What an incredible gift, and one that we can all benefit from when life seems to be too much to handle.

Grit

Grit = courage and resolve; strength of character

In order to climb out of The Pit I also had to embrace my grit. I've always been gritty—I was no stranger to committing to something and really going for it. But those efforts had always been to achieve something. I wanted to be recognized whether it was as a performer in my youth, as a student in my MBA program or as an athlete. I had never used grit to face a situation like getting out of bed every morning in chronic pain or dealing with withdrawal from drugs. I had never used grit to face doctors who didn't believe in my pain, who made me feel like a drug addicted housewife. I was unfamiliar with this particular type of grit and unsure how to use it. And when using grit in this manner, I found there was no pot of gold at the end of the rainbow—no award, no degree, no applause. This kind of grit hurt.

The kind of perseverance it takes to attend hundreds of doctor's appointments, telling my story fifty different times, to fifty different people, with fifty different sets of paperwork is hard to understand. This kind of grit takes a level of commitment and patience I was not accustom to. And in order to harness this grit I had to believe in myself. I had to believe in the pain through the haze of narcotics and the many, many people who did not believe me. And let me tell you something, that was so fucking hard. I questioned myself so many times. Am I crazy? I mean, everything in my life continued to turn upside down no matter how many "good choices" I made and it would get so much worse as time progressed. I had to dig so deep to find a place so raw where I knew in my heart of hearts that what I was feeling was real. And I used that knowledge to keep moving forward.

Even though this grit was painful in its own way, it was grit nonetheless. We all have the ability to harness this quality within ourselves.

People often ask me now what motivates me to keep pushing my limits, what makes me so desperate to return to that strong athlete? Honestly, I don't really know. And it's not even about being an athlete anymore—it's more about not letting my circumstances define me. I didn't want what I had been through to dictate my ability to live a life that was full of movement. I was going to fight for it.

There have been so so so many "first-time afters" in my journey…. first time after surgeries, after hospitalization, after miscarriage, eventually after injections and rejections; first time sitting up, standing on two feet, walking, running, biking, climbing. All of these first times have one thing in common—they took guts. There was nothing harder than knowing I was going to be weak, that I had lost all of my strength, that everything I had worked so hard for was gone. That I was going to suffer over and over to get my life back. But none of that mattered. Accepting that I would never compete again or be able to ride 100 miles on my mountain bike again was unacceptable to me. I was unwilling to give in or give up.

Life Lesson #3 – We are all warriors

I believe everyone has a warrior in them. But everyone's warrior looks different. We're all capable of amazing feats of strength and resilience, but in order to realize our ability to be warriors we must first believe we are worthy of the title. We have to have something in our lives worth fighting for. My warrior may be more visible via accomplishments of endurance or strength, but that doesn't mean that your warrior is any less important just because it can't be measured in miles. A warrior is a person who perseveres under any and all circumstances. By definition, a warrior is a fighter. So, don't be afraid to fight for what means something to you. Who cares if other people mock your efforts and label you "crazy?" They clearly don't understand what it means to be a warrior. And really that is just too bad for them.

It just takes believing in yourself, and making strides in your life that mirror those beliefs. Being a warrior means forming your own thoughts and not accepting anything that doesn't align with your beliefs. It means to fight and display grit for what you know is *your* truth. Without grit I never would have made it through that decade. In the future I will use it in ways I am much more familiar with, but at that point in my life I used it just to get out of bed every day. I use my grit to continue to fight for my life and for the powerful woman I knew was still inside me somewhere.

CHAPTER **17**

My Ladies

I LOVE MY girlfriends. I have always had strong female relationships, but they have ebbed and flowed over the years. I'm not the best at keeping in touch. I am not the woman who still meets up with her high-school friends on girls' trips. I only went to my ten-year high school reunion to show everyone how awesome my life was and check out how everybody looked in their late twenties. I only send out about twenty-five Christmas cards every year and generally don't care if I get any from others. Since I grew up largely on my own, I've mostly been enough for myself. I enjoy my time alone and have never really felt the need to cultivate deep feminine bonds.

And if I must be honest, women can be kind of annoying—always sensitive and emotional. I generally prefer my relationships with men. In my younger years many of those guy friends just wanted to get in my pants, but as I grew older, most of the people I worked with were men and I liked that. Men are generally straightforward and I always felt I could hold my own with them. No tears, deep talks or emotions needed.

Before the birth of Lexi, I had three real girlfriends, one of whom I am no longer in touch with, one who moved to California, and Jen. Jen has been with me through it all and still is my best friend today. She has been my rock and is surely the closest thing to a sister I have ever had. I love her so much and would go to the end of the world for her. I know we will grow old together and someday sit in rocking chairs on the porch of my mountain house drinking wine and smoking weed talking about the good old days. But, before that, we will share mountain bike rides and hikes, backpacking trips with our daughters and countless conversations that only we can have. Talks that only two women who know literally everything about each other can have. We will be brutally honest and tell each other things that no one else will. We will share joys about our children and tears about our relationships. We will share everything. Jen has taught me what it means to always be there. Our relationship hasn't always been perfect and there was even a year or two over the course of our twenty-five-year friendship when we didn't even talk. But that is the true hallmark of a sisterhood—a friendship that stands the test of time.

After Lexi was born I rekindled another college friendship with Taryn. She lived in Denver with her college sweetheart-turned-husband and two beautiful children. Taryn had a difficult time after the birth of her son and struggled with postpartum depression. Jen was actually the one who suggested that she call me. Who better to talk to about challenging babies than me—remember how miserable I was after Lexi was born? I helped Taryn through that tough time, letting her know that she was not alone. That, I too, had suffered greatly when Lexi was born and I let her know her feelings were normal. I also assured her that as time passed she would feel better. Those conversations would lay the foundation for another female relationship that has been with me through my entire journey. It's not easy to be friends with someone who is constantly miserable and suffering, but Taryn never wavered. She was and still is a great listener and a steady part of my life today.

Then there's Heidi. Truth be told, when I first met Heidi a few years before Lexi was born, I thought she was just too intense for me. Heidi doesn't do small talk. So, when you sit down with her, you better be ready for the deep dive. She's going to ask you tough questions and make you think. Back in the early 2000s that kind of conversation didn't really interest me. But as I plunged into early motherhood, Heidi became one of the most amazing girlfriends, one I knew I would have in my life until the end of days. Heidi has taught me what it means to show up. Because in my darkest times, she was there with me holding my hand. She was never too busy for me even though she was running a publishing company and pursuing a master's degree with two kids. Heidi was always there, and I believe that no matter what I need in this world she will be there to bring it to me.

When you become a mom, all of a sudden you have something in common with a lot of other women in the world: you have an offspring. This is an open window for conversation and potential connection. But let me tell you, when your kid(s) are young, every woman has something to say about raising babies and how you should be doing it. As a mom I looked for like-minded women who shared my approach to parenting or at the very least didn't try to tell me how to parent—enter Katie and Erica. These ladies were parents at Lexi's "school" (that's what we parents who send kids to daycare like to call it.) They were both fiery and strong and we immediately connected. Katie was honest and kind, a parent of three and a full-time teacher; she was always pressed for time. But in the summer, we would spend days at the local pool with our kids, dreaming up ideas for our future. Katie would listen hard to my challenges and try—like, really try—to help. When Katie listens, she really listens. I think she honed this skill being an elementary school teacher. The kids could be screaming, thunder roaring and fire engine sirens blaring and Katie wouldn't miss one thing I was saying. Amazing.

I loved Erica for her no-holds-barred attitude to life. Scrappy and crass in addition to loving and empathetic—the perfect marriage of traits. And even though Erica has a high-paying fancy account management job and two kids, she always found time to reach out and check on me. She tells me I am her hero. And I believe she means it.

Lastly there is my suburban housewife posse. By the time Lexi entered our local elementary school I had started to meet and connect with some of the women in my neighborhood—Melissa, Erin and Juli. We plan happy hours, barbeques, camping trips and events in our community. Our kids are quite literally growing up together. I love these women and all the joy they bring to my life. I have laughed so hard with them I peed my pants and I have shared my tears as I struggled through all of my trauma. I connected with them halfway through my decade of pain and they accepted me just as I was—broken. They loved me anyway and they were always there to give me hugs and offer to help with Lexi. They brought me food after my surgeries—some dishes were questionably edible, but all made with love. These three women are incredibly important to me and I hope our connection continues to grow even more as the years go by.

Nine girlfriends (including Keira), NINE, to help get me through all of my shit. And I needed every single one of them. After almost thirty years of keeping females at arm's length, I learned to let them in. And you know what I found out? They are all warriors. Between them and their extended families you will find mental health challenges, affairs, Hashimotos disease, children hospitalized, celiac disease, knee surgeries, foot surgeries, hip replacements, alcoholism and death. These women are fighters with brilliant minds and strong hearts. I am beyond grateful for each of them and their role in my recovery. Each one did their part by reaching into The Pit blindly to help pull me out. Sometimes I gave them my hand and sometimes I let go. But they never stopped trying.

In order to cultivate each of these friendships I had to do something I was not accustomed to doing. I had to give a little bit of myself, I had to be vulnerable and open my heart. And I am so happy I did.

CHAPTER 18

Downward Spiral

I WAS OFFICIALLY "clean" and off all of the painkillers by December 2015, but the pain was still there every minute of every day. I went in for my three-month post-operation follow up appointment with Dr. Peter when he suggested that I try more diagnostic injections. I obliged, but had little faith that they would yield any new information. I mean, was there anywhere else for them to inject? As I expected it didn't work, so I doubled down on my physical therapy, dry needling, massage, etc. in an effort to get better. Dr. Peter said maybe I just needed more time to heal after everything I had been through. "Okay fine, maybe," I thought. I'll keep my life simple, take it easy and hope for the best. Between January and August 2016, I worked diligently to return to a normal life without pain, but I never got there. Things got progressively worse, and eventually I had trouble just walking. I returned to Dr. Peter on August 8 and he agreed at this point in recovery, pain was not normal. He ordered another MRI to take a look at the replacement and promised he would get back to me as soon as possible. The next day Lexi and I headed to Buena Vista, Colorado for our annual camping trip with Heidi and her daughter.

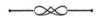

Regardless of my physical health, this annual camping trip has happened every year since our daughters were five years old and is still going today. When we initially planned this outing, Heidi and I hadn't intended it to be a tradition, it just kind of happened. We both felt strongly that we wanted to raise strong, capable girls. We wanted them to know that they don't need a husband, boyfriend or man to go camping and find adventure in the mountains. We wanted to give them the space to roam, make fires, cook, hike and explore. A few days away from the noise of the world is so cleansing and beautiful, but it's hard to believe that if you never take the time to experience it. We wanted to create that opportunity for the girls.

Before I left for the trip Dr. Peter gave me a prescription for Narco (generic Vicodin). This was the first prescription for a narcotic painkiller I had received since taking my last OxyContin. I remember filling that prescription and staring at the bottle in the Walgreens drive-thru. *Is this really happening?* Am I really starting back down this road again? The soul-crushing truth was a resounding yes. For the first time in eight months I found myself taking opioids again. And once again even after all the hell I had been through during withdrawal, I was so happy to wash those pills down my throat and find some sweet relief. Because my tolerance for these drugs was still so high, I had to take two to four 5-milligram pills to dull the pain even a small amount.

Since our campsite was out of cell coverage, I knew if Dr. Peter called I wouldn't hear the voicemail until we drove our car into town. Even though I was trying to enjoy my time camping with the girls, thoughts of what might be wrong plagued me. I mean, something was definitely wrong and I was totally sure of it, but what? I had full confidence that the MRI would tell us the story and then I would be able to assess the situation and decide how I was going to handle it. I was so obsessed with getting a message from Dr. Peter that I drove the car into cell coverage at least a dozen times during our three days camping. But surprise, surprise—his office never called.

I tried to give him the benefit of the doubt, and assumed he had emergency surgeries or some personal family matter to attend to. I mean, he promised me he would call and let me know the results as soon as possible. I had been so upset during that visit to his office, hysterical, crying and snotting all over the exam table. There was no way he could have forgotten about me, right? Wrong. Because you know what, the MRI showed every part of my hip replacement was intact. In Dr. Peter's professional opinion, I was fine. And that, for obvious reasons, did not require a phone call to me. This pain was clearly all in my head.

When I finally got that message from his medical assistant almost a week after my appointment, I was beside myself with grief. What the hell? Of course, I called back and left messages saying he had to call me back, that the results could not be right. That I am in pain, God damn it. Something is wrong.

By the time we left the campsite, my hip had deteriorated significantly from all of the effort associated with pitching a tent, carrying supplies and coolers in and out of the car. I was turning a corner in a bad way. When we got back to Boulder, Heidi had to lend me her family's set of crutches in order for me to walk. I finally spoke to Dr. Peter the following Monday morning, one week after my MRI, when he said, "Sorry, but there isn't anything wrong with the hip replacement and there is nothing I can do for you."

Been there, done that. Heard that before. Okay then, well fuck you, Dr. Peter, I'm going to figure this out with or without your damn help.

Heidi:

This camping trip was symbolic of everything I have ever known about Erin. Erin, she shows up regardless of what is happening in her life. She kept her role as a wife, a mother and a friend throughout her whole process. She never stopped managing appointments, disappointments, recovery and resilience over and over and over. Even though all this was happening during our camping trip, it didn't matter. Erin was great at compartmentalizing. I knew she was struggling, but she kept being as present as possible during this experience with our girls. She let out her grief when it was least hurtful to everyone around her, especially Lexi. Intentionally protecting her childhood for many, many years.

When I found out that Dr. Peter didn't seem to believe Erin, it made me so mad. If they only knew her, I thought. Erin is a fighter and has no issue with hard work. The doctors not believing her was evidence of them not seeing her for her greatest quality. Her drive to be physically strong is like that of a warrior. And even though I sometimes thought she pushed too hard, I knew her pain was real.

At this point, I felt like I had nowhere left to turn. And what do we humans usually do when that happens? Go back to something familiar. I decided to go see Dr. Omer once again. I spent over four hours in his office on August 17. He tried so hard to find the source of my pain. Between his daily load of patients, he kept coming in and out of my room injecting my hip and adductor muscles right there in his office. Usually this kind of procedure is scheduled separately, billed separately and done by someone other than a surgeon. I knew right then and there that Dr. Omer believed me. He believed I was in pain. Unlike the doctors I had seen recently he was willing to go above and beyond. I could tell he was immediately invested in me and even though I had not taken his advice on more than one occasion, he didn't hold a grudge or say "I told you so." He treated me like a real human being with a really big problem. I wasn't an inconvenience to his practice, I was a woman in trouble, and clearly, he cared.

As expected, none of the injections made a lick of difference. And let me just quickly say something about all of these injections—they sucked. And they hurt a lot. When someone pokes you right where you hurt most, it doesn't feel good. And that day Dr. Omer did three or four of these in a row. Ouch! Because of the lack of success with the tissue around the hip, he suggested perhaps I have an MRI on my spine. He thought maybe the problem was not with my hip at all, and maybe we were looking in the wrong place. I scheduled a Spinal MRI for August 30. I would review the results with Dr. Rachel, one of the other specialists at CU Sports Medicine. Fingers crossed, maybe she would have some answers.

But before I left his office that day, Dr. Omer gave me his cell phone number. Did you just read that right? Yes, you did. *His cell phone number!* He said I could reach out to him anytime. That day he promised me he would help me get to the bottom of my pain and I believed him. By this point, he knew that whatever was wrong with me was outside of his scope of work. But by giving me his cell phone number, he was also giving me a lifeline. I was so incredibly grateful that I had found someone who not only believed me, but said he would stick by me. And he did.

Dr. Omer:

I had no reason not to believe you were in pain. I just saw a human being that needed my help. There was no sign that you were a person that was NOT really suffering. I felt I had to do everything in my power to help you.

But truth be told I give my cell phone number to all of my patients. It is the only number they get after surgery. I figure if they are going to trust me with their life and health, I should be their partner through the entire process, not just in the operating room. The difference for you was, you weren't really my patient any longer. I could do nothing else to help you.

Between my visits to Dr. Omer and Dr. Rachael I also decided to see my pain management doctor again. At this point, I couldn't walk at all without crutches and could barely put any weight on my left leg. This was an unacceptable way to live. I think Dr. Lief was disappointed to see me back after I had freed myself from the hold of painkillers less than a year before, but I think he too believed my pain was real, so back I went on OxyContin. Can you believe it? After all of that time and the battle with withdrawal—it was all for naught. Here I was back in the same place I had been a year ago, and instead of needing Oxy to run and exercise, I needed it just to stand up on my own two feet. With the help of the drug, I was able to walk with just the aid of a cane. I was a forty-three-year-old woman with a cane and a handicap sticker on my car and no idea what was wrong with me. I was mortified, devastated and heartbroken.

At this point, the writing was on the wall. I had to take control of my health and in order to do that, it would take my undivided attention. I decided to quit my job. And I had *no* business quitting my job. Our family needed my income. Even though Todd had a great sales job, life in Louisville, Colorado was expensive. And I was also seeing doctors day in and day out, and that was costing a fortune. There had been recent changes in my current employer's business as well and even though she would have kept me around, I knew it was time for me to go.

The next week I had my spinal consult with Dr. Rachael. She didn't find anything remarkable, and only suggested that I do a few more diagnostic spinal injections with another doctor as well as participate in nerve testing. This particular time marked a major shift in my care. Doctors were no longer just looking at my hip as the cause of the pain. There were throwing around terms like muscular sclerosis and spinal/nerve damage, pelvic floor problems, etc. For the next four months I lived in my own personal hell. At least two or three times a week I found myself in various doctor's offices searching for answers, filling out paperwork and telling my story over and over again. On the weekends, I lived in a narcotic haze and prepared for the next week's fight. I was miserable.

Dad:

You need to understand (if you don't already) that what you went through was pretty hard for me to take as much as it was for you to have to suffer through. By no means is that supposed to be a comparison about the severity of it all. It's just a fact from a father's perspective. All throughout your life when those times arose that things might have gone south for you know that I would have done most anything to try to fix whatever might be wrong. So, when I had to watch this horrendous period unfold and was powerless to help, the emptiness was all consuming. This is not the way life was supposed to go. I'm the one who's supposed to get sick. I'm the one who's supposed to need help. I'm the one who's supposed to be operated on. Had that been the case, it all would have been much easier. But it wasn't, was it? All I could do was try to be supportive. *"Things will get better, you'll see."* I>m not sure if I ever really believed that after so many disappointments, *but I wasn't about to quit thinking that it will all end one day and the sun will shine again. It was kind of like that losing season that never ends until it does. There's always next year I'd tell myself, throwing all my efforts into seeing that didn't happen again. If I could do it, so could you. A message I'd try my best to convey. But it was so hard to watch my kid having to endure all this... it just didn't seem fair. She'd done nothing to deserve any of it.*

CHAPTER **19**

Life on Drugs

I GENERALLY HAVE a hard time lying. If you ask me if your butt looks big in those jeans, and it does, I would tell you straight, "yes, yes it does look big." My friends probably love to hate this about me. If they want to know how I feel about something, all they need to do to is ask. Over the years, I have learned to do a better job of waiting to be asked for my opinion rather than just offering it up to anyone in the room. I'm more tactful and have a greater ability to discern appropriate times and tone when sharing something that might be hard to hear.

For example, now if someone asks if their butt looks big, I say, "Well I think these other pants would be much more flattering," or "Those jeans don't have a good cut, they wouldn't look good on a super model." You see what I mean?

But when I was on OxyContin my filter was almost nonexistent, especially when I would add a fast-acting Vicodin on top of the extended-release drug. I said whatever I felt like saying whenever I felt like saying it. I remember being at one of Lexi's "back to school" nights at the beginning of fourth grade. At these events, parents come together in the evening to meet the elementary school teachers and learn a little about the curriculum for the year. After Lexi's teacher was done talking to a room full of parents, she asked if anyone had any questions. There was silence for a couple beats and I chimed in, "Sure doesn't look like it." It was totally inappropriate. The other parents laughed a little uncomfortably. And when they looked at me with that "did you really just say that?" look, I shrugged like, "Yeah, I did, so what are you looking at?"

When my daughter asked me if she was good at singing, instead of saying "Well honey, you sound great singing in the choir, but you might need some practice in your lower register," I said, "No, sweetheart, you're not." OxyContin took away my tact, my empathy, my ability to care about much of anything. And on top of that I didn't care that I didn't care about anything either. It was not just the pain in my hip that was dulled, it was the pain everywhere. I lived in a fog. And the fog was a calm place where I said and did what I wanted. My biggest concern on a daily basis was making sure I knew when to take my next pill. I wanted to make sure that I didn't have to leave this state of emotional and physical indifference for one precious second. Because I knew I would not like my real life one bit.

Don't get me wrong, my physical struggle was real too. I never stopped going to doctors or searching for answers even during my second time on OxyContin, but the only way I felt like I could keep moving forward was on OxyContin. If I hadn't had pain relief, both physical and mental, I would have been suicidal. Deep down, I knew I couldn't be on drugs for the rest of my life. So, one afternoon, lying on my bed looking out the window at the clear blue sky, I decided that if I had to live in pain for the rest of my life, I had two choices: cut off my leg at the hip joint, or die. I couldn't see any other way out. If no doctor could find the source of the pain, I could not live like this forever. I would have to be committed to a mental institution—the pain would eventually drive me certifiably crazy.

The real irony of my life on drugs is I never appeared fucked up to anyone. I drove carpools, attended soccer games, volunteered at school and had dinner parties. It wasn't like I was drooling on myself or stumbling around like an idiot. I seemed pretty normal to most everyone, except maybe my husband and my mom, the two people who spent the most time with me. My mom used to say there was no light in my eyes. Even during joyful periods with Lexi, my exuberance was always muted. There was always a slight distance between myself and any given experience. I didn't smile much, but I didn't cry either. I just existed, day in and day out, moving through life like a good-looking zombie.

Mom

At first, I was in denial. I didn't really know what was going on. I thought it was all going to be okay. The doctor was prescribing the drugs and managing the dosage to make the pain bearable. I felt like it was safe. I always believed that something was wrong with Erin. My biggest worry was that if she stopped looking and the doctors stopped believing, that would be the end of her life. I am crying as I write this because it was just so horrendous. I was more worried for the rest of her life than I was about the drugs. I didn't think she would end up shooting up someday in a back alley. Did she love those pain killers, yes? But at the same time she couldn't wait to be off them, to be whole again.

Todd and I just tried to make it through each day. Truth be told, I didn't think much about him either. He was just the person who picked up the slack when I couldn't do something. I don't think I fell out of love with him, but I couldn't really feel love anymore. I could only feel pain, or nothing at all. We grew deeply apart during these last few years because the stress on each of us was so great, there was no room for much connection or joy. I couldn't even conceptualize sex or romantic relations. Emotional intimacy wasn't something I cared about either and it generally wasn't something I could provide. The distance created by my pain and dulled by the drug would bring us to the brink of disaster years later. But, for now, we were just trying to get through each day. And keep our family together in the process.

And then there was the pooping. It's no secret that opioids cause constipation. So, when you're taking them for years and years, it can become a very big problem. I could not poop without the help of an additional aid, usually in the form of a colon cleansing supplement or a tea called Smooth Move (God, I love that name). That was just a fact. I couldn't take these harsh laxatives every day so I resigned myself to going number two about once every three days. And it was never easy, sitting on the toilet FOREVER just hoping something would come out. And considering I'd had a partial colectomy in the past, this was a potentially dangerous situation. But just like everything else, I didn't really think about it or care that constipation could cause me further harm. I just did what I had to do to poop. End of story.

Opioids also helped me make some very bad financial decisions. Relatively recently I had to admit something to my husband: I had been hiding a $5,000 credit card bill for over three years. I had transferred the balance from one interest-free credit card to another trying hard to pay if off on my own, but having little success.

Then one random morning I was looking for my driver's license and he was going through my wallet when he saw the credit card, one we don't share as a couple. He asked me what it was for and I straight up lied to him, "It's an emergency card, just in case something happened to our other card." He looked at it for a moment and then point-blank asked me, "Does it have a balance on it?" "No", I answered. And then I felt awful... I might have stretched the truth on occasion to my husband about this or that, but I had never told such a blatant lie. Within an hour of his question, I came clean and told him the truth, which was this:

When I was in the middle of all of these tests, this misery and all the drugs, I took comfort in online shopping. I spent hours perusing Nordstrom and Anthropologie websites ordering boxes and boxes of clothing and shoes I couldn't even wear. I have always loved shopping, I mean I am an apparel buyer for a living, but this behavior was completely insane. We had no money because of my constant doctor visits and I had just quit my job! I had no business buying anything, but I just did it anyway. I loved getting all of those boxes on my front door step. It felt like Christmas. Sometimes I would just go on an insane spending spree at three or four different websites and watch the "gifts" show up. It brought me such joy to come home from some horrible experience at yet another medical office to find these treasures at my front door. But with the feeling of elation also came a feeling of shame. I'm not dumb, I knew I shouldn't be buying anything. But like everything else, I just didn't care. I thought that buying stuff would bring me joy, and to an extent, it did, for about two minutes. I was being irresponsible, I knew it, and it didn't matter.

In retrospect, I can look back and understand why I did what I did, but after carrying around that burden for two sober years, I didn't realize the level of shame and guilt I felt. Telling Todd about this debt served as the final barrier to complete truth. And even though on the day I told him I cried for many hours, I am so glad I did and he was incredibly supportive. I think I felt like I needed to carry the burden of the debt as a reminder of how horrible that time was, what a mess I was and what I put everyone in my family through. None of those clothes or shoes made anything better. In fact, they made everything worse. I can see all this clearly now. There is no shirt or great fitting pair of jeans that can make a person happy.

Life Lesson #4 - Happiness comes from inside

Happiness comes from acceptance of where you are and finding gratitude in the moments that test you as a human being. Don't get me wrong—to this day, I still love a good shopping trip. But now I spend within my means and that feels good. I also focus on spending money on experiences and not material things. I'm pretty sure I won't remember a sweater or a necklace over a wonderful getaway to the desert biking with my husband. Experiences fill me up now, not things.

The other night I was watching "Hunger Games: Mocking Jay Part 2" with my family (spoiler alert: don't read any further if you haven't seen the film). It was almost the end of the movie when Katniss Everdeen is lined up to shoot President Snow. She has her arrow pointed at his chest and I am thinking, "NO, she can't kill him. She just can't, that would make her as bad as the rest of them!" I am literally on the edge of my couch and I have NO idea what is going to happen. Then when she points the arrow upwards and shoots President Coin dead in the chest, I am shocked and proud and I think, now, THAT IS a story!

What does this have to do with being on drugs? Let me tell you. Before that night watching the movie with my family, I had not only seen the movie twice, I had also read the book! So how could I NOT know the most crucial detail at the end of the story? Because in many ways, I lost those years on drugs. Not completely—I mean, there are general events or actions I remember. But everything in the middle is pretty much gone. And the details are just not there. Like, I know I read *Mockingjay* and saw the movie, but I couldn't remember what happened. I know I had a birthday, but I couldn't tell you what I got or did for it.

For all intent and purposes, I was taking opioids daily in some form or another from the latter part of 2013 through 2017, finally ending the OxyContin dependency on April 26 of that year. During that time my daughter was five to eight years old. For that entire time, I was there, but not there… When I look back, I think I did a good job being present and participating in all of her activities. I was in her classroom helping out, planning holiday parties and hosting playdates. I never missed anything unless I was in the hospital! But the problem now is I realize that I don't really remember any of it. When I look at pictures sometimes I can't place the event. Like it is nowhere in my head, and sometimes I remember it wrong. It's like a finger-painting in my brain, all mixed up.

And the saddest thing about it, is that I still thought and often think I was a good parent during all of this. But who am I kidding? Really, I was good at faking parenting, at faking everything. Not one person knew the level of dependency I had developed, and developed fast.

OxyContin and opioids take away the color of life. You don't see the rainbow, but you don't see the black either. It's all just swirled together, impossible to separate. For some people this is the allure—nothing doesn't feel like anything. The joy of life is gone, but so is the darkness. Life is hard, and in order to fully experience it, we have to be open to its highs and lows. You can't have one without the other. It is the yin and yang of all things.

Whenever we go on vacation somewhere Lexi is always telling me that she wants to stay forever and I tell her, "If this was all we ever did, it wouldn't be so special. Today would just be like every other day." What makes a vacation so special is actually its opposite. The hum-drum life we are accustomed to is why we feel such joy on vacation. Without one, you can't have the other. On Oxy you have neither, so everything feels the same all the time.

Jen, my best friend:

Did I think Erin was nuts? Sure, but I've always thought Erin was a little nuts. But in a good way, in an amazing way. In a way that Erin would not be Erin if she wasn't a little nuts. That's just her, and it's what, in part, makes our friendship so great! And during this time, when Oxy was her BF more than me. I was ok with that. Relationships naturally ebb and flow—especially ones that span decades. And this relationship was no longer easy. I certainly wasn't giving it up, but was I okay sitting on the sideline for a few weeks? I was.

There were times I felt like I was looking at our friendship through a glass lens.

I remember cleaning out my medicine closet one day and finding a bottle of OxyContin that my husband was prescribed for a knee surgery. Out of 30 pills, he probably took 1. Twenty-nine pills of Oxy is a lot of happiness for someone addicted to Oxy. It felt like I stared at that orange bottle with the childproof cap for several minutes battling with whether or not I should give it to Erin. I didn't.

She was always very transparent with me about how much Oxy she was taking. Well, I thought she was being transparent. But truth is—if she was lying to everyone else around her, odds are she was lying to me too. I was probably getting at least half truths though, and those helped me believe that Erin wasn't a true addict. True addicts don't disclose regularly how many drugs they are taking, right? Was she trying to keep me somewhat in the loop so if things really got out of hand I could step in? The scary thing is that in hindsight, she was at that point. I should have stepped in. But damn it—Erin is good at making you believe what she (and you) want to believe. That she's "got it all under control."

People often ask me if I can take opioids now after everything that happened, and the answer is yes. I can take them and then stop. It's not a big deal for me. I think this is the difference between being an addict and dependent. When I do take narcotics, my brain LOVES them. It's like the Christmas lights go on in my head. My body will always know those opioids. It's like riding a bike. For a while you think you have forgotten how it feels, but as soon as you get on and pedal, everything clicks.

The first time I went to the dentist to have some work done long after breaking my dependency for the second time, he offered me a prescription for Vicodin to dull the pain in my mouth. Just ten pills. Ten gorgeous oval gateways to bliss. Yes, I definitely want those, I thought. And I did. Not just for the pain, but for all the "benefits" of the drug. I took all of them in two days. Could I have gotten by with Ibuprofen, maybe? I don't really know or care.

And that, my friends, is the most messed up part of all. If I could buy Oxy at Walgreens, would I still take it? Maybe…

CHAPTER 20

Dr. Horror

THERE WERE SO many appointments during this time, it's hard to decide which ones are worth writing about. And honestly, any one of these appointments alone would not have been a big deal. But when your full-time job is seeing doctors, getting injections and telling a story no one seems to believe, it's exhausting. So, I'll focus on just three visits in September 2016:

Nerve Tests

In order to test the functionality of the nerves in my leg, Dr. Racheal essentially had to shock me. I was warned it would be unpleasant, but I had no idea how painful it would really be. She put these little white patches up and down my legs and arms. Each white patch had a wire connected to it and those wires were connected to a machine in her office. In order to test each nerve, I had to be shocked. Dr. Racheal would set a frequency on the machine and then send a shock through the wire and into my nerve. And holy crap, did it hurt! My mom came with me to that appointment for support, and I remember her crying, because I was crying. Each shock hurt so badly. It felt like a taser. And because I already hurt so much, it was as if my mind had put up an alarm system. Each time I was shocked I felt it through my entire body. It was as if the shock reverberated from the nerve in my leg to the bottom of my feet to the tip of my nose and everywhere in between. If I was to have this test today I don't know if it would feel as awful. I don't know if I was just so sensitive from all of the poking and testing on my poor body or if those shocks were really so horrible. It doesn't really matter. Everything during these months feels like a nightmare, in fact while writing this section of the book I had to take weeks of time between. It is so hard to go back to this place in my mind.

After the test was over, Dr. Racheal proceeded to tell me there was nothing wrong with my nerves and she suggested I go see one of the hip replacement specialists at UC Health on the Anschutz medical campus in Denver. She gave me two names, another Dr. Michael and another doctor who will remain nameless because I don't want to have to get a lawyer to publish this book. Unfortunately for me, Dr. Nameless (a.k.a. Dr. Horror) was the first appointment I made.

Dr. Horror

This appointment was by far the worst of my entire experience. Take that in for just one second. The WORST of my entire experience, and not because it was painful or long, but because this man made me feel small and lost. Swanky and young, Dr. Horror waltzed into the exam room with copies of my X-rays and MRIs. After asking me to tell him my story, he proceeded to look at the imaging and say, "Well, Erin, there is absolutely nothing wrong with you." And he didn't say this with compassion and empathy. He said it in a matter-of-fact, I am completely sure you are a crazy-ass-drug-seeking-housewife kind of way.

He asked me how long I had been on painkillers, then he asked me if I had a job, he asked me if I had a happy marriage, a happy marriage?!?! What the fuck does that have to do with my pain? I felt so insecure next to his proud, confident demeanor. He stated that he was 100% certain there was nothing wrong with my hip replacement. And, in a roundabout way, told me to "get a life."

My mom went to this appointment with me as well and when we

left, I think we were both dumbfounded. I mean, have you ever had someone say something awful to you and you replay it back over and over in your mind wishing you had said something witty in response? That you had beat someone at their own game? That is exactly how I felt. I didn't defend myself. I didn't stand up for what I knew was real. I had just walked out of the office quiet as a mouse. Dr. Horror basically said without actually saying it that I was a depressed woman addicted to painkillers. And this is the hardest thing about being a person on opioids—you are immediately stereotyped as an addict, or just plainly, a drug seeker. Because I was taking painkillers and there was no obvious reason that I was in pain, it was assumed that I was a girl who just liked her pills.

Dr. Horror is the lowest common denominator in medicine. He did not see me as a person in pain. He learned about my medications and passed judgement. He didn't listen to me. He stereotyped me and then walked away. I cannot stress how unfair this was. Well, I have a surprise for you Dr. Horror, not everyone on painkillers is a junkie. Not everyone on painkillers is a fiend. Many of us are just people desperate for pain relief stuck in a system that doesn't support our challenges.

When was the last time you read about the woman who took painkillers for years and came clean all by herself! You never hear about the person who took drugs so she could be an available mom, so she could volunteer at school and cook dinner for her family. Then this woman goes through withdrawal not once but twice, all by herself. You never hear about her triumphs. Our healthcare system assumes the worst about people and the media feeds it. Well, I am here to tell a different story. I can tell you I couldn't be more grateful to Perdue Pharma for developing OxyContin. I am so incredibly grateful for this drug as it made my life bearable for many years. Is it perfect? No. Are there drawbacks to taking it? Yes, of course. But without opioids, I have no idea where I would be right now. I don't even know if I would be writing this book. OxyContin was a lifesaver for me.

And you know what, I get to say that because this is my story. I don't have to be like everyone else and I get to tell you that there a lot of people like me out there. But they are scared to share their stories because it isn't commercial. It doesn't feed the media drama. Because in the world we live in, people like to hear all the bad stuff, all of the bad in the world. But for every horrible story revolving around OxyContin, there are as many tales of good—you just never hear them.

That visit to Dr. Horror did something else to me that day—he made me question my myself. When I left his office, I thought for a minute that maybe he was right, maybe I didn't hurt. Maybe it was all in my head because of my dependency on opioids. Maybe all I wanted were more drugs and maybe I would be like this for the rest of my life. He broke me down that day, he scared me. He made me feel like I was crazy, like I didn't matter. And to this day, I hate him for that. I have often thought about writing him a letter and saying "see, you asshole, I was in pain, I was broken and you didn't believe me." But I have never done it. Maybe because it hurts so much.

I am 100% sure he doesn't remember me, but I will never forget him. And when this book is published I will hand deliver him a signed copy with these pages dog eared, I guarantee it.

Pelvic Floor Therapy

Another working theory at the time was I might have a pelvic floor issue. The pelvic floor is the muscular base of the abdomen and is attached to the pelvis. When it gets very tight, like any muscle, it can be very painful. I was referred to a pelvic floor physical therapy clinic for an evaluation.

In order to access the pelvic floor, the PT sticks his or her (in my case it was a her, thank God) hand up your crotch and feels around. Quite honestly, by this time nothing really phased me anymore, so, fine whatever, poke around up there and tell me what you find. Again, the therapist discerned there was no indication of any problem with my pelvic floor. Struck out again.

CHAPTER 21

Pin Cushion

OCTOBER 2017 WAS diagnostic injection month. Once again, I was injected so many times, I lost count.

The first was a sacroiliac (SI) joint injection. According to SpineHealth.com, "sacroiliac joint dysfunction is improper movement of the joints at the bottom of the spine that connect the sacrum to the pelvis. It can result in pain in the low back and legs, or inflammation of the joints known as sacroiliitis." Well I certainly had inflammation of the joint, so it seemed like the injection could be a good option. It was done under ultrasound and required that I check into the hospital. I hated those injections the most—the ones where I had to drive to some hospital, wait in the waiting room because doctors are on time about 10% of the time, fill out more paperwork and sometimes the SAME paperwork I had already filled out somewhere else, wait some more, disrobe, change into hospital dressing, all so they could stick one needle in me and ask "can you still feel that pain?" And the answer was always yes, I can still feel it. This time was no different.

Next was a femoral nerve injection. The femoral nerve is the major nerve supplying the anterior compartment of the thigh. It runs from the top of the pelvis to the mid-inner thigh. I did often have pain centered in the groin area, so the working theory here was perhaps the nerve was compromised and causing discomfort. Todd had to drive me to this appointment because I was told I might have a little trouble walking afterwards. The actual procedure was quick, then Todd drove me back to the house and dropped me off. Before he left for work, he helped me upstairs to the bed where I was told to lie down for about thirty minutes. Then I was to try and stand up to see if the numbing relieved any of my symptoms.

After resting for the prescribed number of minutes, I sat up in bed and tried to stand up. When I did my left leg completely collapsed—my knee buckled and I crashed to the floor. Stunned, I sat there in silence and thought, oh my God, did I break something else? I mean, I CRASHED to the floor, my left leg was completely paralyzed. I couldn't move it whatsoever. I had to pick it up with both hands and straighten it out. It was one of the most frightening moments of my life—to try and stand up and then fall to the floor. I was petrified and shaking, trying to recover some composure in order to assess the situation. After doing an evaluation with touch and sight, I decided that nothing additional was broken. I slid on the floor out of my bedroom and down the stairs. I continued sliding on my butt to the living room couch where I used my triceps and right leg to push myself up on to a comfortable seat. And there I lay for eight hours, until I could feel my leg again.

And you know what the most ironic part of this procedure was? My hip pain never went away during this whole process. I couldn't feel a thing in my entire leg, but my hip, oh hell yes, it still hurt.

The Pudendal Nerve injection was one of the final attempts during this month of injections. In fact, I had a series of injections just the day before this one. Dr. Lief, my pain management doctor, was going to perform the procedure and he was running very late that day. Again, I had to check into the hospital and go through all the "check in to the hospital crap" first.

Dr. Lief thought approaching this nerve could be a possible solution, not necessarily for diagnosing my pain, but rather to just help me be "not so miserable" on a day-to-day basis. The pudendal nerve is the main nerve of the perineum. It carries sensation from the external genitalia of both sexes and the skin around the anus and perineum, as well the motor supply to various pelvic muscles, including the male or female external urethral sphincter and the external anal sphincter. At that point, I was willing to do just about anything to help curb the pain. The doctors did not want to give me anymore Oxy, so I felt like I just had to keep fighting.

When I got into the procedure room, it felt strangely like an OR— really cold, bright lights, everyone dressed in surgical garb. Usually when I head into an OR I'm about to be knocked out unconscious and it all seems quite surreal. But this time, I was way too alert. I was scared.

Dr. Lief asked me to come in and lie face down on the operating table. I was naked under the gown and he asked me to open up the back to expose my rear end. Then I was told to put my face in a cradle that had a small opening where I could breathe. There were several nurses around me and I was told to try and relax, that this would probably hurt. I tried so hard to remain stoic and calm. *I can do this*, I thought to myself, *I can do this*. But the minute the needle picked my skin, the tears started streaming and I could do nothing to stop them. They were coming in droves. Snot poured from my nose on to the floor below me. The pain from that needle burned me from the inside. The pain in my hip escalated to a point where I had to cry out. A guttural, primal scream of hopelessness and despair. I just can't do this anymore...I thought, *I just can't*. I was a pin cushion, a voodoo doll.

When it was over and I was able to compose myself enough to stand up,

Dr. Lief asked, "how does it feel?" and I could see the hope dancing in his eyes.

I stood up and put some weight on my left leg. "No different," I answered.

Then I put my head down and hobbled out of the room with my cane.

I entered a new low after that injection, beginning to feel a real sense of hopelessness for the first time. I had been so laser-focused on finding answers, I had quit my job and put my heart and soul into the quest for truth. But I was running out of places to turn, and wondered if I would always be in pain. If I would always walk with a cane. At the time, I really didn't even think about being an athlete again, I just wanted to walk. I wanted to stand up without feeling daggers in my hip. I wanted to be happy. I wanted to stop taking all these drugs. I wanted my life back.

With still no answers in sight and my pain continuing to escalate, Dr. Omer—still the only doctor who still seemed to believe me—introduced me to a diagnostic specialist at UC Health, Dr. MK. The latest theory based on the lack of results from the injections was there could be a problem with my bones, like an unidentified stress fracture. Dr. MK was going to help guide me through a bone scan on November 4. A bone scan is a good way to view and document abnormal metabolic activity in the bones. It's also used to identify if cancer has spread to the bones should that be a concern. This procedure lasts four hours from start to finish. Meeting Dr. MK was like meeting a long-lost cousin or sister. She was kind, empathetic and a great listener. Dr. Omer thought we would get along well and he was most certainly right. Not surprisingly, the bone scan didn't reveal anything remarkable. Because of this and the fact that Dr. MK had never injected me personally, we scheduled a consult and another series of injections on November 22, the day before Thanksgiving. This is another day I will not soon forget. I drove to Denver and Dr. MK greeted me with a warm hug and led me to a room dedicated specifically to her diagnostic injections.

She injected me six times under ultrasound that day and again something just broke inside me. I am not sure exactly what caused this particular breakdown, but enough was enough. The Oxy couldn't protect me any longer from the emotional toll this was taking on me. I was just done; done, done, done. Done with my life, done with the pain, done with it all. Toward the end of the injections, which were all very painful, I just lied there on my back, tears streaming down my face on to the tissue paper covered pillow. Once the tears started, I could not stop them. I cried through the rest of the appointment. I cried when Dr. MK hugged me goodbye and I could see tears in her eyes as well as I walked away.

MK:

I felt, in a word...horrible. In many words, I felt frustrated and disappointed and sad. I wanted to cry.

My thoughts during your first visit were 'what else, what else, what else.' I tried to identify the closest structure to your pain but with every injection...nothing, no change. I didn't want to put you through anymore because with every negative injection response, I could feel your heart break. There are very few times in my life that I felt someone's cry in my soul; this was one of them. I believed you because I could feel your emotional pain and frustration. I felt your cry. After having worked with patients with pain for over ten years, I suppose you just know when it's real.

I stayed in the lobby of the hospital for over an hour crying so hard I couldn't even drive myself home. There was no joy in my heart that day. Just darkness and the blackness of The Pit. I felt so alone as I watched people mill about the hospital all of whom could see I was a hysterical mess. But no one stopped or said anything. I just cried and cried and cried until my tears had literally run out.

That night after pulling myself together I wrote this email to Dr. MK and Dr. Omer:

"Hello doctors,

This week is a time when I always try to reflect on what I am most thankful for. The first thing that comes to mind is family, friends, shelter, food, etc. But this year it is doctors like you that have me feeling incredibly grateful.

I have seen probably 30+ doctors throughout my journey. And I have never had someone care as much as you. Omer, you have stood by me through everything. And MK, you gave a real hug today and that meant so much.

I really believe that both of you care about me as a person, a human being, not just a number or another case that no one understands. I believe that you want to help me and you won't give up as long as I don't. And that, I assure you, will never happen.

So, I just wanted to share my feelings and let you know that you are making a difference in my life and for that I am eternally grateful."

Somewhere between the appointment that day and home I clearly found something special—my resolve. Somewhere between all of those tears and bedtime, I found ambition. Somehow, I found the strength to continue searching and I found gratitude. I found a nugget of truth in all of the mess. That I had people in my life that were fighting for me, that believed me, that loved me. I knew then and there that I was not going to give up. I was not going to lie down in The Pit and be buried alive. I was going to dig deep. I was going to keep pushing.

Dr. MK and Dr. Omer were all in with me too. And on December 22, 2016 we found our first glimmer of hope.

CHAPTER 22

Breakthrough

MK DECIDED WE needed to go directly into the cup of my hip replacement because the doctors had literally injected everything else. Even though the imaging never suggested that there was anything wrong with my bionic parts, MK had her suspicions. She did the lidocaine injection while in the process of having a Computed Tomography (CT) and following the injection she put three cubic centimeters of air to illustrate the flow around the margin of the cup. What she found was that the metal cup had not adhered to my pelvis and air was able to pass through. For some reason my pelvic bone never grew over the replacement cup, meaning every time I stepped on my left leg, the cup was moving ever so slightly in my pelvis, causing the unyielding pain.

After the injection I wrote this email to MK and Dr. Omer:

"I haven't had any pain since I left the hospital. I walked to get coffee, sat in the car, came home went for a 1/2 mile walk and made brownies. I have minimal narcotics in my system. This is it! Thank God..."

Dr. MK:

That email was one of the most memorable moments of my career. I honestly couldn't believe it. After the first round of injections and your follow up email, I was mad and frustrated and determined.

I had a long conversation with Omer and remember saying "I tested EVERYTHING. It has to be in the hip." My initial thought was that you might have some indolent propriobacterium infection at the underside of the cup which is why I suggested the biopsy. The thought of injecting lidocaine was to try to confirm that the cup was the problem. Walking into the CT room, my fellow asked "so....why exactly are we doing this?" and I just shook my head...this was a Hail Mary.

This was amazing, awesome, fantastic, unbelievable news. But now the question remained—why did the cup of my hip replacement not "seat" correctly in my pelvis?

There were a couple of working theories:

- I had some sort of allergy to the metal in the replacement
- There was an infection in the joint
- And my theory: the day the replacement popped out and I went to the hospital in an ambulance...was the beginning of all of this.

During the CT injection, MK took a specimen of my tissue so she could send it to the Mayo Clinic where they would test it for strange infections. We had to wait two weeks to get the results. The doctors at the Mayo Clinic were going to take the tissue sample and attempt to grow several different infections over a few days. I had to be patient, but man, I was so desperate and so excited. I knew the source of my pain was in the hip replacement itself. And now I was ready to be done with all this.

Regardless of the cause of the pain, it was determined that I needed a hip replacement revision, which is basically a whole new replacement. That's when MK introduced me to the other hip replacement specialist and head of orthopedics at UC Health, the other Dr. Michael.

Dr. Omer:

Truth be told, I was so happy when that injection worked because MK and I had been Sherlock Holmesing the problem trying to find a needle in a haystack. But most surgeons didn't see a hip replacement revision as the unequivocal answer. Most who did not know you personally were not super confident that another replacement would solve the problem. You were suffering from a bad reputation. From the 30,000-foot view there are many people that fall into narcotic use and we all (doctors on staff) needed to accept that this might be the problem with you. That you won't get better. MK and I were sure, but others were not.

About six months before my appointment with Dr. Michael, I had written a timeline of events and given it to all of my new doctors. It outlined all of the surgeries, injections and doctors I had seen. I thought it would be helpful for these professionals to have a snapshot of what they were dealing with when I walked into their office. I usually emailed the timeline or brought a printed copy to my appointment. I thought maybe a doctor would see something in it and go "ah-ha, I see what's wrong here..." But that never happened. In fact, this new Dr. Michael was the *only* doctor I know who actually read it because he referred to it in our appointment and I was floored. No one had ever read that document—no one. Sure, I had seen doctors take it and put it in my file. But I never saw anyone actually read it and none of them ever mentioned it during my appointment.

As the head of ortho at a major hospital, Dr. Michael was very busy. But the staff was able to move some things around and get me in on February 21, 2017. Finally, I was going to get to the bottom of everything.

When the tests came back from the Mayo Clinic, they were negative, so no infection, which left us all scratching our heads. So, Dr. Michael suggested a surgical allergy panel. I had never heard of such a thing, but apparently you can go to an allergist and they will test you for negative reactions to all things that are used during surgery.

I made the appointment for the following week. To administer the test, the allergist pin-pricked my back about fifty times and then added tiny bits of solution to the holes. After that he covered the pin picks with tiny Band-Aids and sent me on my way. I had to come back the following day so he could assess my reaction to the fluids, and then again three days later for the same thing.

After both "readings" he concluded that I was severely allergic to nickel. I never got any data about how much nickel (if any) was in my current replacement—it didn't really matter. At least the doctors knew that moving forward any metal in my body needed to be absent of nickel. And this time surely that would be the case.

At this point, my left leg was almost completely useless. I could barely put any weight on it without sending spikes of pain through my body. I couldn't even lift it to get in the car. I had to use both hands to pick it up and place it under the steering wheel to drive. I had begged my pain management doctor for more Oxy many times, but he wouldn't budge. So, I started to redistribute my pills throughout the day to maximize my pain relief. I took 20 to 30 milligrams three times during the day and just 10 milligrams before I went to bed. Because lying down was the most comfortable position for me, 10 milligrams was plenty for pain relief during the night. But because I had so little opioids in my body during these hours, I started to go through acute withdrawal, every single night. Once I went to bed, my body was desperate for more narcotics. I was so dependent on those drugs the thought of being without them even for a few hours was terrifying. I often woke up in cold sweats tossing and turning, waiting for the morning sun to come up so I could take another pill.

Dr. Lief did however prescribe 5 milligram tablets of Vicodin. Those were for the worst of times. But quite frankly every day was "the worst of times." One time, I asked Todd to hide the Vicodin from me so I wouldn't take all of them too quickly. I thought if I had to ask him for pills that would make it more difficult for me to take too many. That lasted for about one day, before I tore the house apart looking for the prescription bottle while he was at work. I found it in a storage bin in the garage and promptly downed two Vicodin (in addition to all the Oxy) and waited for the dullness to sweep around the edges of my mind and body.

Because of my drugged-out state, the surgery was a blur. I remember being in the hospital and being in a lot more pain after the operation. But I had a ridiculously high tolerance to opioids, so in order to manage the pain post-op, I became like the walking dead.

When Dr. Michael came to visit me in the hospital, he gave me the socket of my old replacement. You can see clearly the bone had never adhered to the metal, meaning every time I stepped on my left leg the whole thing was moving in my pelvis. No wonder it hurt so bad! Dr. Michael never really told me what he thought about the first surgery or why I was in this situation. Maybe it was because he didn't know, but I believe he had his suspicions too. There is this unspoken rule between doctors, medical device reps and others in the medical community—they don't seem to ever rat each other out. Someone did me wrong somewhere along the line, but by the time I was getting the second replacement, I did not really care. I just wanted to be better. And what would it matter anyway? I wanted my life back and that was ALL I cared about.

Once again, I moved into my parents' house for a few weeks while I started to recover. Since this was surgery number nine, I knew exactly what I needed. I had my own "bring Erin's family dinner" calendar all set and ready to go. My friends all came to visit, some of them for many hours and others for just a few minutes. But they all came because I told them how much it meant to me. The most memorable of these visits were from my friend Kiera. Even though she lived almost an hour away from my parents' house, she came to visit me twice a week and walked with me around my parents' neighborhood. These walks were really just fifteen to thirty minutes outside moving. I had a walker which I relied heavily upon. The walker made travel doable, albeit very slow. I was so thankful for those walks and now they make up my most fond memories of that time.

Keira:

Surgery after surgery, I knew Erin had to be struggling mentally more than she let on in casual conversation. Having meals cooked and helping with her daughter or light housekeeping was helpful, but when you're down and out nothing beats time with a good friend. When your spirits are low, you become apathetic and start letting go. In contrast, when your spirits are high, you take action. It felt natural, to me, to show up, to give hope, to remind her that this was a fight worth fighting. I was happy to spend time with my friend as her spirit transcended her broken body and mind. Walking with her while she limped along with a walker, she demonstrated she was still that tenacious competitor that I love.

It is hard to have people witness your struggle and it is hard to be the one witnessing. When do you give space? When do you insist on showing up? Can you talk about your epic training day or is that rude? Do you downplay all of your struggles because you feel they don't compare to what the other person is going through? In my opinion, all of those questions come down to my own anxieties and insecurities. What my friend needed was for me to show up, be present and offer support and encouragement. It did not feel that different than during our climbing gym sessions or rides or runs.

In July 2019 I got the chance to show up for Kiera just like she had for me. I served as support crew for her 100-mile ultra-running race. Because that is what real friends do. No matter how inconvenient, no matter how challenging, when it matters most—they show up. I was honored to be there to help Keira do something amazing, and I realized a crucial piece of my own story along the way.

In order to provide "support" for Keira's 100-mile running race, I had to be very organized. My job was essentially to coordinate everything Keira would need to complete her journey. I was in charge of meeting her six times, in the six different locations over thirty hours with little or no sleep in between. Travel between each of these encounters included navigating 225 miles of Colorado highways and back roads. At each new spot, I would set up a chair for her to sit down, change her socks, fill her water bottles with water and sports drinks, take away her trash, give her new food for the next several miles, put chaffing cream on her sports bra strap and make sure her pacers (individuals that ran with her after mile fifty) were all set. The unspoken part of my job was to know not just what her body needed, but her mind too. Most notably at mile forty-eight Keira came into the aid station as wrecked as I have ever seen her. I mean, this girl is a beast on the trail and I have never seen much rattle her, especially in the back country. When she appeared around the corner, I started jumping up and down, waving my hands like an idiot. I was so happy to see her and currently she held about tenth place overall. I was expecting to see her pumped up and excited to venture into the second half of her journey, but instead I saw a broken woman. When I asked her how she was doing, she responded through tears, "not good." I thought, oh crap, not good—okay, change of plans.

Then I proceeded to get more information about what was going on in her mind. She warned me that during long races, she can go to dark places, so I was ready. She told me she didn't know why she was doing this, she thought she might be doing long-term damage to her body, and she just felt like stopping. That's when I told her what I knew she needed to hear. That she was amazing. She had let her mind take her to bad places, but she had control over her mind and could change all that. I told her she was halfway there and she was about to crush it (the second half of her races are always better than the first). That this was her defining moment and I wasn't going to let her quit. Then I told her there were four women in the aid station and she better get in there and get her shit together. And you know what, she did. And she totally crushed the rest of the race, getting faster and faster.

In all honesty, I didn't really know what to say in that moment, I just did the best I could and later I came to find out how powerful it had been for her. That I had saved her from maybe quitting. And that felt so GOOD! I had a role in her success just like she had in mine and that made me happy.

Keira:

I have always admired Erin's athletic abilities, both physically and mentally. When out training with her if we saw someone ahead of us she always had a 6th gear to chase them down and drop them. If I had a big objective, she would always encourage me to do it and her belief in me would help cement the idea in my head that it was possible. It got to the point that when training alone, I would find myself thinking of her for inspiration. "Erin would turn it up right now, you should, too." "Erin would sign up for this race right now and figure the training out later. Do it." And so it was that at midnight when the registration for the High Lonesome 100 Mile Trail Run opened, I knew she'd approve of me clicking the "submit" button.

Crewing is a big job and it is hard for me to ask for that kind of help. I knew that she would rather pace me than crew me but I had my sights set for the podium and was worried that the terrain was not suitable for her repaired hip. With lots of experience as an endurance athlete and crew member, I knew she understood, better than anyone, what I would need and not freak out when things got ugly, which they most certainly would. I was beyond thrilled when she agreed to help out and she did not disappoint.

Coming into mile 50 aid station, I felt awful, more awful than I ever had in a race. I was sure that I would drop from the race when I finally made it to the aid station. I had no idea where I was in the race standings but walking felt hard and I couldn't get food or water in me so I continued to spiral downwards. I was being hard on myself for my extreme deterioration, for spending so much time away from family and friends to train "for nothing" and for letting down Erin, my family and my pacers that had selflessly given up their weekend to come help me out.

Feeling like death, I finally see the aid station up ahead and all of a sudden Erin comes jogging towards me with a huge smile on her face.

She is pumped and her energy and enthusiasm a stark contrast to mine. Her face dropped as soon as she saw me. I was honest with her and let her know I was done. Tears started flowing. I felt like a failure. She immediately changed gears from happy cheerleader to diagnostic technician. It was incredible. She took charge, let me know that there were several women at the aid station, that they were not in good shape, that I needed to pull myself together and get back out there. She believed in me and I needed to as well. I weakly accepted that I was not dropping here. I got food and water, necessary night gear and my first pacer and we went off into the night. Throughout the night I picked up my pace, harnessed my inner Erin and passed competitors one by one. I smiled knowing she would be as proud as I was for turning myself around.

30+ hours later from hugging her at the start, I hugged her at the finish. Tears of pain and joy slipped from my eyes. Some say that running 100 miles is like living life in a day. To have Erin witness, support and encourage me throughout that is one of the many things that kept me going in that race and in life itself.

After the race was over, I had more than one person come up to me and say, "if you didn't run with her, what exactly did you do to support her?" They didn't see my purpose, they didn't think I was necessary. I found this fascinating and then I realized something…

People tell me all the time that I am amazing for conquering what I have in the last decade, from doctors to physical therapists to friends and new people hearing my story for the first time. And I can't lie, that makes me proud. But at the same time what about my support system—my husband, my family, friends and doctors? What about them? What about the people who held me while I cried, drove to and from the hospitals, who took care of my daughter, who answered my medical texts at 11:00 p.m. I could easily argue they are the real heroes of my story. Without them, I would not be writing this book today. I would not be sharing my journey with the world and I'd be lost and alone. Without them I couldn't finish the race; without them I'd give up. Without them, I'd never get better.

CHAPTER **23**

Real Recovery

THIS TIME RECOVERY felt a lot different. I mean, I was quite literally building something from nothing. I had not identified myself as an athlete in several years. What would my comeback look like this time? I had no idea, but I can tell you with absolutely certainty, I knew there would be a comeback! There were so many questions swirling around in my brain. What would my goals be now? Would they be any different after nine surgeries? Of course, at first my goals where small—walk without a walker, get off drugs, walk without a cane, walk a quarter mile, ride a stationary bike for ten minutes. There were a lot of baby steps to take and I had to be patient. But ultimately, I knew I wanted to make it to the starting line of another ultra-distance mountain bike race. I wanted this journey to come full circle.

But there would be a lot of ground to cover first.

Dr. Michael told me I could do pretty much anything I wanted once I felt no pain, even run a little. He also told me I would have to make choices around using my new hip. My hip was going to be like a set of new tires. Eventually, it was going to wear out and I would need a new one, it was just a matter of how much I was driving on it. I decided that in order to get back on my feet I would need help—more help than I had ever had before. Not only was I going to PT, I also solicited the help of a personal trainer and my therapist. I had a small army of people committed to helping me get better. I also had a new job! I had been given a one-year contract to purchase apparel again for a single store in Boulder, Neptune Mountaineering. Neptune is probably one of the most iconic outdoor stores in the country and it was right down the street from me. The store had come under new ownership and they hired me to help with the floundering soft goods portion of the business. I was honored and grateful to be given this opportunity. I hadn't worked in almost a year and this job came out of nowhere. It was perfect for me—not too much work, but enough to make some money doing something I loved for a great company.

About two months after the second hip replacement, I had improved enough that I knew it was time to get off the Oxy for a second time and I dreaded it. I was taking about 100 milligrams a day and I needed to get down to zero again. And just like last time, I did not wean myself off at the pace recommended by my doctor, instead proceeding just as I had the first time, reducing my dosage by 10 milligrams a day for ten days until I had no more left. And this time was no easier for me—it was just as horrible as ever.

My first full day without Oxy was a work day. I decided the weekend wasn't the best idea because my family wasn't all that helpful. I didn't really want to come clean about how hard it was to come off the drugs, so I thought the less I saw my husband and daughter that first day, the better. Instead I booked an appointment in Denver to review some apparel choices for the upcoming spring season. I thought if I kept myself busy that would be the ideal situation. I did not, however, anticipate my insane behavior on that day.

The drive to the Denver Merchandise Mart was about twenty-five minutes from my house. When I merged on to the highway that day something very strange happened. It was as if someone had highjacked my whole body and my brain. I pulled all the way over into the Express Toll lane on the left side of the highway and proceeded to accelerate and accelerate and accelerate until I was driving over 100 mph in my four-cylinder Subaru. All I wanted was to go faster and faster. The faster I went, the better I felt. I had NEVER driven that fast in my life. It was reckless and dangerous, but in that moment, I didn't care. I didn't think about the potential consequences of my actions, I just wanted to feel an explosion of pleasure in my brain. And for whatever reason, driving fast was getting me there.

Thankfully, I made it safely to my meeting even though I had no business working in that condition. This was just the beginning of what would be another month of withdrawal misery. The headaches, the nausea, the sleepless nights, the haunting thoughts of The Pit— they were with me all the time. But the one difference was this time, there was no pain. At least nothing like the pain I had experienced in the past. I was getting better and I knew it. I just needed to survive this withdrawal and then I would finally be able to move on.

In late May 2017, I felt something different, something I hadn't truly experienced in so long—real honest-to-goodness hope. Things started coming together. I was drug-free and gaining strength and confidence in my movement. I just knew in my heart of hearts that I was going to be okay. I felt like I needed something permanent to re-mind me of all I had lost and all I had gained through this experience.

In terms of personal style, I have never been an overly decorated sort of person. I'm not big on jewelry or makeup and I can't have my ears pierced because of my metal sensitivity. I love clothes, but not accessories, especially not permanent ones. But on May 17, I de-cided to get a tattoo. I wanted something small and relatively discreet on the inside of my right forearm, a symbol to encompass all I had been through as well as serve as a reminder of what I can and will accomplish in the future. Before I decided on the design I talked to many of my friends about it. And oh my, they were so full of opin-ions. Some said it should say "resilient," but to me a resilient person is someone who gets hit over and over and just keeps getting back up. That certainly defines me, but I am more than just a punching bag or weeble-wobble. Others said it should say "warrior." A warrior is a fighter. And I am that too. But my journey wasn't just about fighting or conquering, it was more about accepting. My journey was about finding ways for me to find joy in all of those awful moments. It was about my spirit rising above the physical pain, accepting where I was and putting back together the pieces of my life. So, I decided on the word "unbreakable" with a dove extending out of the "e". The dove represents my spirit. *Unbreakable Spirit,* now that truly defines me. My body can be beat down over and over, but my spirit can still soar no matter what the circumstances.

I don't think about the tattoo much anymore, but every once in a while, I will look down and notice it or someone else does. And I truly love it. It is a perfect representation of the experience. It is one decoration that I am happy to keep forever.

In June our family took its first vacation in many years. Todd had to work in California, so Lexi and I decided to piggyback on his trip. We flew out early to go to Disneyland! Now let's just consider something for a moment. Five months earlier, I couldn't walk a step without the help of my cane. And now I'm about to walk around Disneyland for an entire day! Nothing could have made me more excited. The first time we did Disney, it was an epic fail. We didn't understand the whole "fast pass" thing. We had tried to wait in line for the rides with our five-year-old in the middle of summer in Florida. It sucked and I actually thought maybe we scarred Lexi for life and she would never want to go back. But lucky for us she had forgotten! This time we were going to do it right. I downloaded the Disneyland app on my phone and first thing in the morning we went straight to Space Mountain and snagged our first fast pass. I have never been so ready to have fun. I was going to walk around Disney for hours and hours and I was going to be just fine.

Lexi and I rode every ride we could that day. We got Mickey Mouse ears, ate ice cream and screamed on roller coasters. We watched the parade sucking on giant lollipops smiling from ear to ear. This was the first time in so, so long I remember having fun. When we got back to the hotel I laid in bed with a satisfied smirk on my face. Wow I thought, this is what matters, this is what I have been waiting for, this is what life is all about. God, I was so happy that day. I was so in love with my husband and my daughter. I was so grateful to be walking and living again. I thought, finally, I have done it. It's over. I am going to be okay.

Movement and exercise now had a place in my life again too. I was going on bike rides and hiking with friends, strength training and starting to feel a little more like my "old" self. But I had no illusions of what I was capable of during this time. Coming back to athletics was a slow burn, and I had to face some harsh realities along the way. I was petrified to ride my mountain bike. I was so scared of falling and hurting myself, I could barely ride at all. I was in a constant state of panic. Rides that used to provide the perfect escape from the drudgery of a work day made me incredibly uncomfortable. I got off my bike to walk on only slightly technical sections. At first, I was okay with it, but after a while I realized it wasn't that much fun to always be walking your bike. I couldn't really figure out what I was doing out there on the trails anymore. I felt like I didn't belong. So, I decided to focus more on hiking and riding on the road. These activities felt less threatening, and I was fairly sure I wasn't going to get hurt doing them.

Then on July 9, 2017, I was reminded that everything was dangerous for me.

CHAPTER 24

Please, no…not again…

IT WAS A typical summertime Saturday in Colorado, bright yellow sun against a cloudless blue sky—perfection. Jen and I were planning a hike in the Indian Peaks Wilderness west of Boulder. We got up early, hoping to be motivated enough to summit the 13,000-plus foot Mount Audubon. It was about a seven-mile round trip and would serve as my longest hike to date since the second hip replacement. I was so psyched to be out there. Being able to move through the woods on the trail again filled my whole soul with joy. It wasn't often that Jen and I could get out for a whole day, so it was an extra bonus to be up there with her. And everything was going our way. The parking lot at the Brainard Lake Recreation Area is notoriously crowded. It is almost impossible to find a spot even when you arrive at dawn, but on this day that was not the case. A family had just finished their hike when we rolled up in Jen's car. Neither of us could believe our luck. It was shaping up to be a great day.

And it was, for miles and miles. I couldn't remember the last time I had been up that high in the mountains. Up above 11,000 feet there are no trees, just rocks, scrub, sunshine and wind. It was chilly, and the temperature dropped as we rose higher and higher to the base of the scree field just below the summit. We certainly weren't the only ones up there that day, but our journey was extra special. I was elated to have made it to the top. My hip was holding up and felt relatively strong on the hike. To be honest, I was a little more scared about the descent. It was going to be hard for me to descend 3,000 feet back down to the car, and I wondered how my new hip would fair by the end of the day. We took it slow as we made our way back down into the trees. And my hip was really sore, but it didn't hurt in a bad way. Just in an "I am ready to be done walking now" way.

Then about a mile from the car, I fell.

But it wasn't my hip that gave out, it was my right ankle. It just collapsed under me. I hit the dirt with a thud. Stunned, I grabbed the flesh around my ankle bone as it seared in pain. If you have ever rolled your ankle you know this pain. Often you can shake it off and it's no big deal, but other times it can be debilitating for weeks if not months. Shocked and dumbfounded I looked up at Jen. She looked back at me equally baffled. What just happened, I thought? Clearly, I had rolled my right ankle—not good, but not the end of the world either. Hopefully I was going to shake it off and keep hiking. I moved it around in circles in both directions, then I flexed and pointed it several times. It hurt, but I was able to move it without hearing any loose parts wriggling around in my foot. We weren't far from the car, so I figured I could get there, get home and RICE (rest, ice, compression, elevate) and everything would be fine. After about five minutes of catching my breath, I stood up on shaky legs. Then I took maybe ten steps when it gave out again and I crashed on to the trail. This time it was worse, the pain was stronger and I was scared. Never in all my years of rolling my ankles had it EVER happened twice on the same hike or trail run. These were unchartered waters. I could tell that Jen, too, was worried. I pulled the first aid kit out of my day pack and proceeded to wrap my ankle with an ace bandage. Now I was worried and I started to shake a little. The adrenaline coursing through my veins made me light-headed. It had been only five months since I had received my new left hip and here I was falling on my right ankle. It literally seemed impossible that this was actually happening.

After a few minutes on the ground, I stood up again with the ankle firmly wrapped and took a few more much more tentative steps. It seemed like the wrap was going to help provide the support I needed so we continued on toward the car. Less than a quarter mile later, it happened again! It was like my right leg was saying, "I have held you up for the last four years and that was long enough." I am done. I give up. I quit. My ankle was like jelly, ligaments and cartilage loose and moving around under my skin.

I burst into tears. *No, no, no, no, no, no this can't be happening.* This CANNOT BE happening. I have to be able to hike. I have to be able to move through the mountains on my feet in some way. I had lost my ability to run, but I could not lose the ability to hike. This was not okay. I was not okay.

After that third fall, Jen let me drape an arm around her shoulder and she quite literally carried me to the car sobbing like a baby. I was horrified, hysterical and petrified about what this meant for my recovery. I knew first and foremost I needed to get to the car and then I would need to see my ankle doctor for an evaluation. I knew something was very wrong. Damn it. I had come so far. I was so close to climbing out of that Pit when once again my foot slipped and back down I slid into the darkness. The day was so overwhelming. I went from being incredibly joyful on the top of my first mountain in eight years to crying uncontrollably on the way home as my ankle swelled to the size of a grapefruit.

Once I got home and shared the news with my family, I think they were as shocked as I was. I lay on the couch again, ankle propped up on a pillow wrapped in ice. I tried to lose myself in the television, but my mind was spinning like a hamster wheel. What would this mean for me? What would happen now?

The evaluation with my doctor went as expected. There was severe ligament and tendon damage. He said it would heal up over time, but the injury would likely continue to give me grief and limit my abilities to hike or climb in the future. I wasn't ready to sign up for another surgery so I waited a few months to see if I could get to a place where I could move "well enough" and be happy. But that destination never materialized. Sadly, my right ankle was never the same after that day in July. I had to wear tennis shoes almost exclusively to create the support needed to hold myself upright. And my ankle continued to give out randomly and I would crash to the ground while walking in the grocery store or at home. I knew it was going to need to be fixed—I couldn't live like this forever. So, on December 14, 2017, I scheduled my tenth surgery.

Jen, my best friend:
It's important to understand a little bit about what it's like to be Erin's BF from her BF's perspective. Erin (by choice) keeps her circle small and tight. But if you are in that circle, she would literally give you a limb if you asked for it. It's also worth noting that while Erin and I play outdoors a lot together, our exercise relationship is very different than, say, Erin and Keira's relationship. Erin handily kicks my ass in most exercise outings and it's always been that way. I don't have the competitive drive she does so it's never affected our relationship, but it has created an image of her in my head of a warrior.
Erin hiking to 13,000 feet a few months after a complete hip replacement would not come as a surprise to any of her friends or family. Our hike up the mountain that day just reiterated every thought I've ever had about her: she is relentless, she is persistent, she is (as her tattoo states) unbreakable! But is she?
As we neared the car, I believed the section of the trail Erin first fell on was probably handicap accessible (or if not designated that way, certainly could have been). It was as smooth and as flat as trails in Colorado come. We were casually strolling at this point, our feet starting to hum as they knew the car was within reach, and then all of a sudden I heard a thud and turn to find Erin on the ground. Honestly, the first time she fell I turned around and thought, "What in the hell is she doing on the ground? She just climbed to the top of a mountain. She's obviously not really hurt. She's Erin. She's invincible." So, I helped her up and we quickly brushed off the incident. Perhaps we

both wanted to pretend it didn't really happen. And then, in what felt like seconds later, THUD! She's on the ground again. Now a dark and harsh reality sets in. This isn't good. I'm looking at my BF, my friend who can literally conquer anything she puts her mind to. But I'm seeing a fragile soul in a puddle on the ground. A soul that is literally at its breaking point. We both assume once she wraps her ankle with the Ace bandage, that would certainly get her back to the car. But after the third and final time of falling within a fifteen-minute stretch on a flat surface, we both fell silent. Eventually I did what any BF would do—tried spewing all sorts of positive thoughts like "your strong, it was just a little too much, a little rest and it'll heal"—but in my mind I'm running the gamut of thoughts ranging from she really WILL be fine, to will she EVER be fine?

This operation would essentially mirror the left ankle surgery from 2012. My doctor would go in and attempt to reattach the ligaments and repair the damage. My ankle would be non-weight-bearing and immobilized in a cast for six weeks, then I would have a walking boot for another four weeks and then physical therapy and recovery. This surgery is a long road. I remembered that from before, but I promised myself I'd be strong and survive. That everything would someday be okay and this was my path to walk. Why, I hadn't the faintest idea—but here I was going under the knife yet again.

After the surgery was complete, my doctor said there was quite literally "nothing to work with" in my ankle. He had to use synthetic pieces to string everything together. I knew he did the best he could, I just hoped it would be enough. I also had to take post-surgical painkillers again. No OxyContin this time, but still it was scary to put any opioids into my body. I didn't know how I was going to react. Turns out I still enjoyed the pain relief coupled with indifference, but the addiction I beat almost a year ago did not rear its ugly head again. I was able to take the drugs and stop without much trouble.

The fact that I wouldn't be walking for over a month, and that all of my weight would have to be supported by my new hip, was nuts. Just nuts. I think even after I had the surgery, I was still stunned: WTF!?! And it showed up in all aspects of my life. I was short-tempered, cold and generally pissed off, mostly at my husband.

Todd had been such a trooper through all of my ordeals, but after this last surgery he was stretched too thin as well. His coping mechanism often involved drinking maybe a little too much, and one night it all just blew up in our faces. I know he felt sorry for me, but at the time, I didn't feel sorry for him. I was just wallowing in my own self-pity. Blaming my unhappiness on my situation, I was sure I was never going to be whole again and I was truly broken somewhere deep inside myself. I didn't think the dark cloud that had followed me for a decade would ever go away no matter how much positive self-talk I generated. The brewing conflict came to head one night when I suggested to Lexi that Todd was drinking too much and that was why he was acting (like an idiot)...such an inappropriate thing to say to your child, but I didn't care. I wanted him to hurt like I hurt inside. I wanted him to stop being okay with drowning his sorrows in beer. The relationship had become toxic and I think we both knew it.

Truth be told I had resented Todd for years. Over the decade that I was in pain and dealing with these numerous setbacks, Todd had continued to ride his bike relentlessly, getting faster and faster. He started racing the ultra-races I used to race. And I went to support him. But when I was there, I was so sad—life didn't feel fair. I wanted to be racing, that was the way it was supposed to be. I didn't want to be his support, I wanted him to be my support. But what I didn't realize then is he had been my support, for years. He took care of Lexi and me through so many bad times. He was loyal, compassionate and always showed up. Maybe he didn't cope with his feelings as well as he should have, but hell, we all make mistakes and errors in judgement. I didn't realize all this for many months after my tenth surgery, so that night when we were fighting things got as bad as they ever have. I was so mad...I screamed at him that I hated my life and everything in it. And then I threw my crutches at him right in front of our daughter. A lot of damage was done to our relationship that night, and it had been heading in that direction for a long time.

Not only had Todd flourished on his bike, but he also had grown exponentially in his job, receiving at least three promotions and spending a lot of time at work. With these promotions came more travel which was also difficult to navigate with all of the surgeries. The resentment built to a crescendo that night and I knew it would be a long time before we healed. In reality we didn't deal with our issues for many months. We just coexisted in the same house, two people raising a daughter we both loved very much.

About six weeks after the surgery, I had to attend an Outdoor Industry trade show in Denver. It was imperative for my job. The show was held at the Colorado Convention Center and included all relevant outdoor brands. The show requires that buyers walk between vendor booths to view products, sometimes covering as much as three to six miles a day. I had to do this on crutches! No, it wasn't the first time I have had to "walk" a trade show on crutches, but this was by far the hardest. My body was just so tired from all it had been through. I was exhausted.

The time I spent crutching around the convention center yielded a surprising new change in my body—I lost feeling in my right arm. Yep, you read that right, my arm. I had never had any problems with my arm before, but after crutching through the show for three days, a whole new issue surfaced. And once again, I was scared. I could not feel my hand or fingers. It was like I had sat on them for twenty minutes and got up. You know that tingly feeling you get when a body part "falls asleep?" It was exactly like that, but the prickly feeling did not go away. I went to a hand doctor who suggested that perhaps I had carpal tunnel syndrome, so I went in for an evaluation. Thank God, the results were negative. The hand doctor thought I had most likely created the numbness with pressure under my arm using the crutches to cover so much distance at the trade show. He didn't know how long it would last, but hopefully it would resolve itself over time. I was relieved to hear this, but at the same time it wasn't definitive. All I could do was wait and hope.

Part Four
Healing

CHAPTER 25

The Warrior Spirit

POST RIGHT ANKLE surgery was a bad time for me. Starting another comeback story seemed fruitless. I felt like a pretender, a hoax. I thought there was no way for me to ever be okay again, until I met Melissa, who I had been referred to her by one of my more spiritual physical therapists. Melissa is a Shaman. The word *shaman* means "a person regarded as having access to, and influence in, the world of good and evil spirits, especially among some peoples of northern Asia and North America. Typically, such people enter a trance state during a ritual, and practice divination and healing." And even though this normally would not have been my cup-o-tea, I was eager to try anything that might help me turn a corner.

My first meeting with Melissa was unremarkable. I knew nothing about her and she really knew nothing about me. She asked some basic questions and then did some "muscle testing" where she pushed on my arm or elbow and took "readings" of what was coming up. She wrote the findings down on a form. Here is what she said and I have added my own thoughts about the specifics in parenthesis:

1. Betrayal/Abandonment, at or around the age of thirty-five. This felt like a work-related relationship. (leaving Running Specialty Group)

2. Anxiety, at or around the age of twenty-five. (moving to Colorado)
3. Feeling of dread or blame towards self or another after the age of thirty to either present or within the past five years. This felt like a close relationship, I think your husband. (Having Lexi and then what I just described in the previous chapter)
4. Feeling of being unsupported after the age of thirty to present (through everything)

I thought this was pretty spot on. When she did the testing, she said things could come up that might be way in my distant past. But I didn't really have anything overly painful happen in my distant past. Everything was relatively recent, and that showed up for her as well which I thought was interesting.

She also asked me if there was something I was looking for in our meetings and I told her that I was really struggling to get better both mentally and physically. I told her my body and mind had been through a lot and I felt like I couldn't break the hold depression had on me even though I was still taking anti-depressants. I told her the truth—I was seeing her because I didn't know what else to do.

She told me she would meditate on this idea and ask her "guides" how to proceed. She explained that her "guides" were spirits that helped her access and process the issues of others. She said we all have guides but very few of us know how to communicate with them. She told me that they would help her better understand my situation and how to address it. This is what she wrote to me via email after that meditation:

"So, when I went to ask my Guides…He said that (that there was a) conversation with your Self that occurred, (when that happened) it was like a little seed was planted. But, this wasn't just a 'seed of doubt', it was a seed of *hopelessness*. And, it took root in your heart and now has tendrils reaching also into your mind. He said that it was this seed that was keeping your body from accepting the healing that you've tried to give it. Like, someone who's convinced that the sky is purple, and no amount of showing them otherwise will change their belief. Think, a stubborn two-year-old who has an idea in their head and just won't let it go no matter how ridiculous. This has nothing at all to do with logic. The Heart is all about feeling, not logic.

He said that this seed could be removed and he showed me how to do this (which we did), and in its place, we planted a seed of healing, love and hope. He said to draw this energy not from *my* Self (which is how we normally do things), but from the child you. That 'pure' childhood hope that we all remember having before we learned about disappointment. It was like filling a tiny little bucket with that pure, intense hope and happiness, and then carefully carrying it back and planting it in the hole that had been left by the Hopelessness. Once that was done, the tendrils of that same doubt and lost hope were removed that were going up into your head. It was interesting, because it wasn't as deeply rooted in your brain as it was in your heart.

In moving forward, his main suggestion was that you hold yourself in love and let this take some time to work. That you treat yourself with the same compassion that you would show your very best friend who just had surgery or some injury…

(In addition), there's something in shamanism called the 'fractured soul', and it can occur when something tragic or upsetting happens. It can also happen over years of a chronic illness or suffering. It's not like split personality though. It's like a part of your spirit just can't deal with something anymore and it sort of shuts down from the rest and breaks off and then kind of gets lost. I think there's an element of that going on here, too…it's very possible to relocate that part and once it's integrated back into the whole, then that can also help the healing begin to pick up and move a little bit faster.

Curious to hear how you're doing today. And I'm sure you have a ton of questions. Again, sorry this sounds so weird. Sometimes the 'weird' is unavoidable and to try to make it LESS weird would lose too much in the changing :)"

What? This was crazy—I mean this woman did not know anything about me and here she was talking about my seed of hopelessness. And when I read her email, it made me cry. It was like I knew it was true, at some point between that hike up Mount Audubon and recovering from yet another surgery, I became hopeless and the feeling had engulfed me. I was living in a place of continued blackness and I wasn't sure how to pull myself out anymore. Practicing gratitude seemed pointless and continuing to step up and rise above my situation seemed impossible. At the time I really believed I would always be broken.

Nonetheless, I was encouraged by her words and her plans to help put together my fractured soul. The truth was, I felt broken not just on the outside, but on the inside too. Even though I was hopeful Melissa could help me, I was still skeptical of this actually being "real." Even though I was impressed by her ability to nail down some of the lowlights of my life, putting my soul back together just seemed a bit improbable, if not impossible.

Then on February 25, 2018 I became a believer.

When I got up that day I felt nauseous and sick. Unable to focus, I was irritable, generally pissed off and on the verge of tears all morning. In itself this wasn't that uncommon for me, but for some reason, on this day, it felt different. Like something deep inside myself was off. It was incredibly unusual for me to not be able to relax and focus in my yoga practice, but that morning I was just a mess. I couldn't put my finger on it until I got this email later in the day from Melissa:

"How are you doing today? I just wanted to double check that you did alright yesterday and last night and see how you're feeling today.

...Like we talked about, soul retrieval is the process of finding pieces of our Self that have somehow gotten lost. When we find them, they often look the age that they were when the event occurred, so if in childhood, the piece looks like a child. For you, this particular piece was (again) in your mid-thirties, and I apologize in advance if this is too personal.

...The piece that we found was sitting outside in a wooded area. She wasn't crying, but she was stuck in the state that she was when she left. She said, "He's going to leave me. He's going to leave me...because I'm never well. I never feel better when he asks, and he asks all the time, and I know it upsets him when the answer is no. I'm not going to feel better ever. And he *should* leave because it's never going to change.

I told her that he hadn't left. That he'd stayed and so had her daughter because they both loved her. It took a lot of convincing. At first, she said she wanted to come back because she (wanted to) make him feel like she did. We made it clear that wasn't necessary anymore, that her daughter was getting big and that she was happy. That things were different now and all that mattered was that they stayed and that they loved her. All she had to do now was go back and feel all of that...She agreed to come home. We delivered her to you and she's now a part of you again.

I'd like you to pay close attention to how you're feeling today. Sometimes the integration process can bring up some emotions that haven't been dealt with because those emotions left with the piece that broke off...some of the emotions might not make any sense because you can't pin them on something that just happened...

Let me know if you have any questions. The only thing you really need to do at this point is to be gentle with yourself...You're doing a great job. I hope you slept okay and that you're not having too bad a day today."

WWHHAAATTTT?????

When I opened this email and read it, I was floored. She had given me an explanation for what I was feeling that day and I was 100 percent sure in that moment the soul retrieval was the cause. I just "knew" it. I felt it in all of my being from the bottom of my feet to the top of my head to the pit of my stomach. It was everywhere. And

I thought, "this woman is for real." Over the next week I felt a wave of relief and a new clarity about my healing. Slowly, the clouds in my brain started to part and I could see a brighter future.

After this experience with Melissa, I thought I would see her a hundred times. I was so happy with the results and so excited about the idea of her continuing to refine my soul. When we first started together she told me that people only see her usually four or five times. Then they often stop because they "get what they need." I couldn't believe it—why would anyone stop wanting this feeling? I mean, I felt remarkably different and was certain it would just get better and better over time. But sure enough, I only went one additional time after the first soul retrieval piece. I can't explain why either. I just didn't go back and we didn't keep in touch. She was right. I had received what I needed, and I was good. Even better than good—I was hopeful and ready to start finding myself again.

And the first place I can always do that is on my bike. I wasn't allowed to ride outside yet, since it would have been too difficult to get in and out of my clipless pedals with my newly reconstructed ankle. So, I put my bike on the trainer in the basement and just started pedaling again. It was hard and boring. I committed to a few Netflix shows and downloaded a new "comeback" playlist on my iPhone and just started to spin.

Music has served as an external motivator for me for many years. When you spend literally thousands of hours riding your bike on endless mountain roads, it can get quite boring. Don't get me wrong, the Colorado scenery is breathtaking and beautiful and I appreciate it all the time. But having some hardcore music that moves you pumping through your headphones on a steep mountain pass—well, that is just the bomb.

We all are motivated by different sounds, beats and voices. For me, it's hip-hop. Rap music has always been my jam. Not sure when it started, probably dancing in St. Louis. I took ballet, jazz and even tap for a number of years. But it was hip-hop that spoke to me. Sometimes I like to think I was Black in a former life. I feel so connected to the music and the movement of African and urban dance. And I love it. It's fraught with passion and delivered with "a chip on the shoulder." And I feel like I get that, now more than ever.

I love it when people look at me even now and they are like, she's forty-seven years old, she can't do that.

She's had ten surgeries, she can't do that.

She's been out of the game for so long, she can't do that.

You think I can't?

Well, watch me.

Granted, there is some rap music that doesn't resonate with me. I am not a big fan of overly derogatory lyrics. It's the beat and often the message, it just makes me want to move. And move hard, whether it's dancing, riding my bike, or just bobbing my head in the car. I can't stop it. I feel like my body is wired to embrace it. I can't really explain it better than that.

I knew I would have to start somewhere and sometimes starting is the hardest part. I also decided to register for the Telluride 100-mile mountain bike race that would take place in late July 2018. That was only five months away, but why the hell not? If I didn't show up, I didn't show up. But there was zero chance I would show up if I didn't register in the first place. I liked having a goal and I figured why not pick a big one? I knew I wanted this journey to come full circle, but I wasn't sure I could actually do it. But that didn't really matter at the time. The race gave me something to think about and that was enough. I made a collage of magazine clippings like the ones I used to make in seventh grade. It had words like "goal," "be better," "break the mold," "power" and "strong." I taped it up by my bathroom mirror so I had to look at it every day. It was a reminder of where I wanted to go. It was a reminder that I was going to get better and today was the first day of the rest of my life.

Sometimes committing to a goal like that, especially one you are not sure you can accomplish, can be really scary. I had signed up for this race twice before, but never made it to the start line. What would make this year any different from those years? I really didn't have an answer. But I was sure of one thing—I was going to get up every day swinging. Every day would be about getting stronger and focusing all of my energy on recovery and strength.

And not just strength in body, but strength in mind. If I was going to compete in another ultra-distance mountain bike race, I would need to refine my mind. The defeatist mentality I had been embracing would need to shift. I would have to believe reaching this goal was actually possible. I had to believe it every day, on good days and bad days alike. I would have to show up every morning for my family and for myself. I would have to work harder than I had ever worked and I would have to be okay with whatever outcome my body gave me.

Riding my bike was not just about riding my bike. It was not about getting fit enough to compete again, it was about so much more. It was a metaphor for everything in my life that I had lost. Each time I tried something for the first time after recovering from that last surgery, it was a gamble. I never really knew if my body would hold up. I was petrified of getting hurt again and each step outside my comfort zone felt enormous. At first, I wouldn't get on a trail. I would only ride on the road and only on flat terrain. I rode tentatively and with caution. Each thirty-minute or hour-long ride felt like one small step toward healing my spirit. Each time I arrived home, I felt a sense of relief. Okay great, I made it, I'm still okay. I can do this. It was one baby step after another, and as my confidence grew, my body healed.

Then one day in May something remarkable happened. It was one of those bluebird Colorado days and I headed out on my mountain bike. There is about twenty miles of single-track trail right outside my backyard in Louisville. It isn't technical or difficult, but it's fun. I hadn't ventured out there since I had been cleared by the doctor to

ride, but today was the day. And as I pedaled through the familiar terrain, I was overwhelmed by a sense of gratitude for being able to be
out there again. And I realized for the first time in as long as I could
remember, I felt good. Like really good. Like my old self good and
I just started crying and laughing and crying and laughing. I took a
selfie on the trail of my broad smile and tears streaming down my
cheeks. For this was the first time in so very long they were tears of
joy. Pure unadulterated joy.

And then the remarkable kept happening...over and over.

One morning I rode to the top of Flagstaff Mountain. Five miles
straight up, and when I got to the top, I had to decide—do I roll over
the other side and commit to another three hours of mountain riding
and climbing, or do I go home where it's safe and I know I will be
okay? I sat on the top of that mountain for about ten minutes. Should
I do it? Could I do it? What would it cost me if I did? But if I didn't roll
over the backside of that mountain, I would never know. If I never
gave myself the chance, I would never see what I was capable of. I
knew in my heart that I was ready, I could do it. I also knew it would
hurt and I would suffer. But this was the good kind of suffering. This
was the kind of suffering I was born to do. So, I did it.

I plunged down the backside of Flagstaff and breathed in the crisp
spring air. I was going to do it. Not just on this ride, but on every ride.
I wasn't going to let anything get in my way. No one was going to
tell me I wasn't going to get better, no one was going to tell me I was
some drug addicted housewife, no one was going to beat me down. I
was going to fight and claw and push, because that is who I am. And
that day I knew for sure that nothing would stop me. I was taking back
my life and it was going to be better than ever. I wasn't just going to
survive addiction, pain and hopelessness. I was going to beat it down.
I was going to put The Pit so far behind me, I would never see it again.

CHAPTER **26**

Redemption

IN ORDER TO prepare for the Telluride 100 race, I entered the Breck 68. A sixty-eight-mile race through the backcountry of one of my favorite mountain biking destinations, Breckenridge, Colorado. I had competed in the Breck 100 three times before pre-body implosion, so I knew what I was getting into. This race was the absolute hardest of the 100 milers I had competed in. I knew it would be a good test of my fitness. The 68-mile course consisted of two loops rather than the three for the 100 miler. The first was by far the hardest with the most single track and three big climbs. The second loop was longer but the climbing was less steep. I knew if I could survive the first loop, there would be a good chance I could finish. And to finish was the goal. Actually, to survive was the goal.

Two weeks before the race Todd and I went up to Breck to ride the first loop so I could see how I felt. It was a terrible day. It took us over five hours to get through the ride and by the end, I was completely spent—exhausted, ready to pass out, spent. Todd was like "come on, let's just do the first climb on the second loop," and I thought there is no way. I was a bit defeated that day. I knew if it had been race day, I would not have made it to the finish line. And this scared me for sure. But I had come too far to be deterred. I reasoned that I was borderline over-trained (again) and what I needed was rest. I knew this was a possible cause of my lackluster performance, but I wasn't completely sure anything would be different when we came back.

On the way home that day, we got a call from my parents (who had been watching Lexi). They said she had been injured at Ninja Warrior practice. Her coach let us know the injury was serious. So we went straight from Breckenridge to Avista Hospital.

Lexi discovered Ninja Warrior like most people, by watching the television show "American Ninja Warrior." On the show adults compete against one another on an obstacle course with a series of challenges, and the person who goes the farthest, the fastest, is declared the winner. A certain number of people from each "stage" move on in the series to compete on increasingly difficult courses where they continue to have a chance to move on to tougher obstacle races. The last person standing is crowned champion for the season.

Since Lexi could walk she has always been a very active child. Todd and I enrolled her in just about every activity under the sun: soccer, basketball, climbing, biking, horseback riding, swimming, dance, gymnastics, etc. We looked for a physical activity where she not only excelled, but that lit her up. A sport that made her smile, that she couldn't wait to do. But even though she enjoyed a lot of these activities and arts, she never really cared much about them. She didn't care if she went to class or not. It was something to do and that was good enough.

When Lexi was eight she expressed an interest in Ninja Warrior. I bought a Groupon online for a gym called Warrior Challenge Arena and within five minutes of watching her in the class, I knew we had found her future passion. Lexi's smile was the biggest I have ever seen it. She glowed with a light and brightness I hadn't yet seen in her eyes. She fell in love with obstacle course racing that day and hasn't considered another sport since.

Pulling up at the hospital emergency room that day gave me pause. I could feel the panic rising in my chest as we walked through the sliding glass doors. It was like my body remembered coming to this emergency room so many times, and the idea of being anywhere near a hospital made me physically ill. I had to stop and remind myself that I was okay and needed to be there for Lexi. She needed her mom.

When we entered her hospital room, our sweet little girl was a mess. She had just recently been cast on the first season of the TV show "American Ninja Warrior Junior." We were supposed to fly out to Los Angeles for the filming in just three short weeks, and here we were in the hospital! The doctor took an X-ray of her leg and it was broken. Her dream of competing on the show was over. She cried more that night than I have seen her cry in her entire life. She was completely devastated. And the worst part about it was, I knew exactly—I mean, exactly—how she felt. And it crushed me. Lexi ended up with a full leg cast and was heartbroken.

But after all of the tears were shed, she started to do something I did not expect. She started talking about what she could do right now, in this moment, to stay strong. She asked if she could train with her coaches even though her leg was broken. And I said yes. She told me she wanted to go to Los Angeles and cheer on her friends that were competing. And I said yes. Then she told me she would make her own comeback, this injury would not define her. And in that moment, all the fighting I had done was worth it. Every single time I had to crawl up from the depths of my hell, my little girl was watching. She knew that bad things happen to good people who don't deserve it. She also knew that there was no quitting in our family and it would be no different for her. So, for the next three months Lexi trained in the gym with her coaches. She swung on ropes, rings and monkey bars with her full leg cast dangling underneath her. She did push-ups, sit-ups and pull-ups. She climbed at the climbing gym with one leg just like I had done years before. And even though it was hard and frustrating, she didn't give up. She kept working and fighting because she knew from watching me over and over that this, too, would pass. She would heal and compete again.

Over the next year she would make it on the podium again and again. Proud does not begin to describe how I feel about my daughter. I feel more than proud, I feel honored to be her parent. Wise beyond her years, Lexi is an inspiration not just to me, but to her coaches, friends and teachers.

Today she is thirteen and still competing. Her love for the sport is deep. It has taught her so much about hard work and resilience. Since she started, Ninja Warrior competitions have popped up all over Colorado and the United States. There are several leagues operating on a national level and Lexi has had the privilege of competing in most of them. I have no idea how long it will last, but I feel so blessed that she has been able to have this sport and community in her life.

Armed with her full leg cast, Lexi and our whole family (my mom, dad, Todd and I) headed to Breckenridge on July 13, 2018. Todd was racing as well, so my parents had agreed to watch Lexi while we both had our day out on the bike. Of course, this took on new meaning with Lexi's new limitations, but they were still willing to come. When we arrived in town I had to register for the race, so I wandered over to the race start. A banner advertising "Breck 100" hung over the finish line and as I gazed up at it, I was overcome with emotion. It had been THIRTEEN years since I had started this race and here I was again. I could not believe I had made it this far. I had no idea what would happen the following day as the gun went off and I headed out for an adventure on my bike. But I knew I was strong enough to start, and that alone was good enough for me. I was brave enough to try. The "old" me (the pre-ten surgeries me) would have never started unless I thought I had a chance to win. This was all new. Starting this race took a new kind of strength and a new kind of brave. And I loved it. I loved that I could see life through a different lens now. I could see this race as an opportunity for growth and challenge, but it had nothing to do with winning. I was taking a chance on myself and hoping I would be able to finish and not "die" along the way.

The weather was perfect the next day for the 9:00 a.m. start. All kind of nervous, I could barely get the peanut butter bagel down my throat and I probably had diarrhea five times that morning. I had not felt those pre-race jitters in so long, yet they came back so easily. My body and mind remembered this feeling of angst, they were no stranger to it. I just wanted to get going.

I knew I just had to ride my own race, go my pace and hope for the best. Butterflies littered my stomach as I waited patiently for the race start. Everyone was there including Lexi and her cast! When she hugged me for good luck, I felt her slip something in my bike jersey pocket. She told me it was a note and I should read it later in the race. I agreed. That moment held so much for me—I knew she wanted me to be successful as much as I wanted that for myself, but what if I wasn't? What if I couldn't finish? What would I say, how would I handle it…I just didn't know. And luckily there wasn't much time to think about it, because minutes later it was GO TIME.

Even though ultra-races start out crowded, they thin out rather quickly and then you're out there more or less on your own with your thoughts. As I pedaled through the first loop I tried to stay calm and work at my own pace. As the climbs went by I started to feel tired and then I started to question myself. Why am I out here? What am I trying to prove? Wouldn't thirty-two miles be enough, why do I need to ride 68? Hadn't I come far enough already? Why do I need to do this race at all? But as the toxic thoughts raged in my head something else happened. I started passing people, lots of them. Lots of men suffering on their bikes watching me fly by. I even saw one of them cheat the course and I thought, seriously, at what cost did he need to succeed?

And as I hit the descent down into the transition area where I would pick up fresh supplies for loop two, I got that second wind. I thought, "I can do this, I can really do this." I just had to get in and out of the aid station quickly and keep moving. When I rolled to a stop at mile 32, there was nobody there to welcome me. I went straight to my cooler, filled my water bottles, grabbed food and then I thought, the NOTE! I reached in my back pocket and there it was, the most uplifting thing I could have ever asked for:

"Dear mom,

I am so proud of how far you have come. You are my hero and my inspiration. You can do this. I know you can.

I love you, Lexi"

And that was it. I was going to complete this race if it was the last thing I did. I folded up the note, headed out on lap two, and began an arduous 2,500-foot climb up Boreas Pass. But I had new energy and new resolve. I had finished the first lap in a little over four hours, so I was making good time and I knew I was just going to get better and better. Legs churning, breath steady, headphones blasting my hip-hop; I was in the zone. I crested the top of the pass and headed down one of my favorite trails. I was flying. The perfect marriage of talent, grit and flow right there in that moment, and I knew nothing was going to stop me. I weaved through the forest with determination and pride.

The last climb of the race is always the hardest and that day it was no different. I knew I just needed to keep pedaling. *Just keep going,* I thought, *just keep turning those legs over and you will finish.* There was no one cheering me on, no one there who knew my story. It was just me, alone with my mind. I thought about all of the doctors, all of the tests, all of the pain and all of the drugs. This bike race, ha!, this bike race was nothing compared to what I had overcome. This bike race was just a symbol of what was possible, of what the human spirit can accomplish if given the chance. And as I crested the top of that last climb and sailed toward the finish line, man, that was something. It was all worth it. I had proven something amazing to myself and to my little girl—that anything is possible, you just have to believe. You can never give up because this feeling, this feeling right here, this is what it is all about.

At the finish line my whole family was there to welcome me and I was so happy. I did it. And I wasn't sure if I could, but I had taken the chance. I had made myself uncomfortable, and I had grown as an athlete and as a human being. My daughter grabbed a hold of me, balancing on her one leg and crutches, and gave me the biggest hug. She said "Mommy, I am so, so proud of you." That day was everything to me. I will never, ever forget it. I said this journey would come full circle and I would finish an ultra-distance race and damn it, I did.

Dad:

As to the ultimate triumph in the bike race, well, I've got to admit, that was pretty great. There's an old saying that I used to remind myself of when times got tough in coaching. "What doesn't kill you will ultimately make you stronger." Finishing that endurance race kind of defined that for you. I always knew you were tough but this just kind of defined just how tough! It represented defeating all the trauma you had to cope with over all those years. You may have been down, but never out. I imagine you doubted that day when you crossed the finish line would ever come, but it did. Your perseverance paid off. You never gave up and, in many ways, it sort of opened a new chapter in your life. In the end, I knew you could do it. After all, my kid wouldn't settle for anything less.

In two weeks, the next stop would be the Telluride 100, but first I had to take my one-legged daughter to Los Angeles and attend the Outdoor Retailer trade show…

CHAPTER 27

Growth

THERE WAS A lot to pack into two weeks and it was really more like ten days. Lexi and I left for Los Angeles on Saturday, July 21 and returned July 24. Then I had to attend the trade show from July 24-26. And after that I had to pack all of my stuff for the eight-hour drive to Telluride on July 27 because the race started at 6:00 a.m. on the twenty-eighth. It makes me tired just thinking about it.

Clearly, I had a problem. Well, it wasn't clear to me then, but it is now. After overcoming a decade's worth of health problems, I was obsessed with packing stuff in my schedule and pushing limits. And not just my physical limits, my limits on everything. I felt strongly that I had not been the best version of myself for a long time. So, I was going to be super mom, super consultant and super athlete all at once. I was not able to objectively see what I was doing. I was trying to make up for all of those lost years in one summer, and it started to take its toll on me.

By the time I was driving to Telluride I had a bad feeling. My spirit deflated, part of me wanted to just forget the race, turn around and drive home. The mountains felt ominous and looming instead of welcoming on that overcast, rainy day. And I was tired. I mean, really tired. Still just six months out of the last surgery, I had pushed so hard since then, and now I could feel it all catching up to me. But I was committed. I was committed to start to race, but somewhere deep down I knew that maybe things were not going to go the way I had planned. But just like in Breckenridge, I knew I was strong enough to start, and that had to be enough.

By the time I reached Telluride the clouds had parted and there was a buzz in the air. Racers from all across the country had gathered in this mountain town to experience the event. I waited in line to pick up my race number and pumped the men around me for information about the course. The pre-ten-surgeries me used to approach every new ultra-distance mountain bike race the same way, as an adventure to unfold while I was out there on my bike. I had always made it a point to NOT pre-ride the course, so I could experience the journey fully. I loved watching the trails, climbs and descents manifest in front of me. It was part of the allure of the distance. But that was ten years and ten surgeries ago. Why I thought I should approach the Telluride race the same way, I have no idea.

The men I chatted with in line were sand-baggers—someone who acts like something isn't really that hard when, in fact, it is. And I learned this rather quickly on the first climb of the race the following morning. The guys had said the race "wasn't that hard" and the climbs were "not that big" and the course was "fast." I asked them to compare the race to some of the others I had ridden in, like the Leadville 100, and they said it was about the same. Now granted, I had completed that race sixteen years ago, but it was my first ultra. Somehow, I felt that balanced everything out. Okay, I can do this.

After getting myself situated I found a place to eat some pasta and went to bed. I slept rather fitfully that night haunted by prerace jitters. So, when 4:30 a.m. rolled around I was ready to get this party started. The race would encompass two very big loops. The elevation profile showed two big climbs in the first twenty miles. After that we would ride on undulating single track until we came back through town to retrieve our supplies for the final sixty miles, which looked to be much easier.

At 5:40 a.m. I rolled down to the start line with my cooler and food for the final lap and stashed these goodies, along with extra clothes and bike maintenance tools, for the final section of the race. It was a glorious morning. The rain had left behind cool mountain temperatures and a baby blue sky.

After the race gun went off, I felt a new sense of excitement about the day to come as we pedaled through the quiet Telluride streets. There is nothing quite like knowing you are capable of riding 100 miles on your mountain bike. That's a long way and the path was about to begin. I was excited, heart thumping, as we headed toward the first climb of the day, Black Bear Pass.

I had not studied a map of the course, only really the elevation profile. I knew the climb was steep, but I really had no clue what I was getting myself into and as we started to gain altitude I felt calm and ready. My body seemed to be responding to the effort in the beginning. But as the miles dragged on I realized that this gritty four-wheel drive road was getting more and more difficult. Now, I may not have had the technical skills I once had on the mountain bike, but I was still no slouch either. This "road," if you can even call it that, became more rutted as we got higher, with giant potholes and big rocks the size of large dogs littering the riding line. The grade of the climb also became steeper, and eventually I had to get off my bike and start walking. And let's just get this out of the way, at the time, I was not a hiker. And my body, especially my hip, did not like pushing my bike up a mountain road at 12,500 feet. Especially in mountain biking shoes, which are stiff and not made for walking. It sucked. I was in this race to RIDE my bike a hundred miles, not push it a hundred miles. I'm sure there were some very strong riders who were able to ride this section, but from where I was in the race, everyone was walking. The energy it took to try and pedal far exceeded that of just trudging up the pass on two legs.

I probably walked my bike one to two miles up the pass all together. By the time I got to the top my hip was screaming at me and we had only gone a total of seven miles—*seven* out of a hundred. And that made me very nervous. Those seven miles had already taken a big toll on my body, and honestly, my spirit. At the top of that climb, the first seeds of doubt were planted.

As we descended down the backside of the mountain, the temperature became a big factor. Climbing up I had shed most of my layers and was creating an enormous amount of body heat, but when I stopped pedaling the thirty-degree temperature started to settle in and I got very cold, very fast. The road down was also technical but not as challenging as the climb up so I was able to gain some speed. But with that speed also came the wind chill factor. The breeze stung my face like a thousand tiny pin-picks, my hands grew numb and my teeth started chattering. The dirt road eventually led to a paved section of the course. I went screaming downhill as fast as possible so I could just get to the next climb and warm up. By the time I got there, I couldn't feel any of my extremities and I started to get nauseous.

I pulled over at the bottom of the second climb, Ophir Pass, to pee behind a tree and try to collect myself. This next climb would take me back up to 11,800 feet and over to the town of Ophir. I was way out of my element here. I had no idea where I was in relation to Telluride and I thought if something happened to me, I would be in some serious shit. There was no cell service and very few people were staged along the route. There was nothing I could do. I knew that regardless of my discomfort level, I really had no choice but to keep going.

As my legs began to spin again I started to warm, however, the bile churning in my stomach did not dissipate. I found this a bit alarming so early in the race, but I hoped it would resolve sooner rather than later. This climb was MUCH easier. Even though it was steep, it was not technically difficult. The road was as smooth as sandpaper and just that fact made the whole race somehow seem more doable in that moment.

I climbed swiftly up the pass. And as I crested the top and peered over the edge, I could not believe my eyes—the route down the backside was not a trail at all. It was literally a boulder field. Thousands of rocks ranging in size from a beach balls to zebras snaked down the mountain. You could see an outline of a "road" but it was barely visible in all of the rubble. What I saw before me was steep and dangerous. I was like "oh my God, how am I going to get down?" I cursed myself for not learning more about the race and not coming to pre-ride some of these hard climbs. I was an idiot. One wrong move and I was toast. Once I started down the pass, there was no stopping. If I tried to stop on the boulders there would be no place to put my foot down. The ground was unstable like waves on the ocean. And if I braked too hard or went too slow, I would likely go over the handle bars. I had to trust my bike and trust my skills to survive this descent. I mean that is exactly how I felt, like I only needed to survive. I could not bear another injury. I felt sick. I was way out of my league and there was nothing I could do about it. It was only about three hours into the race and I felt like I had been out there all day.

Deep Breath
In, Out
You have no choice
Deep Breath
In, Out
I started to roll. Gripped.
Don't stop
Don't stop
Keep moving
Don't stop

I have no idea how long it took me to get off that section, but I can tell you when it was over, I was done. My whole body and mind were completely depleted. Eventually once I got to the town of Ophir things started to look up. The rest of the loop was relatively easy riding, just a lot of miles. My stomach was upset as well and I had to stop on a few occasions to poo or actually, have diarrhea, which is more accurate. When I got to the transition area at mile forty, it had taken me six hours to get there and I was about to miss the cutoff. This was BY FAR the slowest 100-miler I had ever ridden. I told myself not to stop…just "get your shit and get out of the aid station. Just keep going." And I did.

With fresh supplies I headed up the climb from town to the ski resort. I knew it was the last big climb of the race. I also knew that I had to ride another sixty miles. Best case scenario, it would take me probably another six hours, putting my finishing time at around 12-12.5 hours. Twelve hours on a mountain bike at altitude is no joke, and just six months out of my last surgery, I was unsure what it would cost me to finish. As the climb started to materialize, my legs felt good while I was pedaling. But sadly, once again the grade became too steep for me to ride, and I was going to have to get off and push my bike again. The first few steps told me the whole story. My hip and left leg were done, revolting with every footfall. I knew it was time to throw in the towel. Could I have finished the race? Yes, probably. But I wasn't willing to accept the consequences of doing that. I didn't want to be so crippled after the hundred miles that I could not get back to my hotel room. I did not want to feel pain for weeks after, and I felt certain that would be the case. I had gone through enough pain for one lifetime. This suffering could actually hurt me and it just wasn't worth it.

I turned my bike around, coasted back down the hill to the start/finish and let the race directors know I was pulling out.

I was quitting.

And honestly, I was completely fine with it. I gave everything I had and it wasn't enough. But I knew I had grown leaps and bounds that day. I had pushed myself out of my comfort zone and conquered many challenges in those six hours. It was enough for me. I went to a bar, had a beer and burger and went to sleep.

The next morning, I could not wait to get home. I left Telluride early and stopped in Como to do the third loop of the Breckenridge 100 race again—it's one of my favorite rides. I felt amazing that day. And I had no regrets about quitting the race the day before. This is what I wrote on my Facebook page:

"Well...this time I can't say, I did it! I didn't...This body has been through enough and I know my limits. And you know what, I'm so good with it. I am so incredibly proud of how far I've come. And no one, no race can take that away. I'm awesome. And I know it."

CHAPTER **28**

Repair

IN THE WAKE of the Telluride 100, I felt accomplished but also a little lost. I had put everything I had into training for those summer races, doing my job and making a great, epic summer for Lexi. In doing that I exhausted myself, and also forgot about the single most important human being in my life—my husband.

Todd knows me really well. And he knew when I was attempting to pack all of these activities and travel into one summer that I was going too hard. But even though he shared his thoughts with me, he also knows I am painfully stubborn and not likely to listen to him anyway. I am going to do what I want. It has always been that way. And deep down I think he kind of loves me for it. But I'm sure it's also quite annoying. Todd likes strong, capable women. I often find him watching women's sports stories on Redbull TV late at night. He loves a powerful female and a comeback story, both of which I certainly am. The problem for me was, at that point, he had never told me that my story was the greatest story of all. He never really told me anything.

Let's back up a second.

And just so you know, this is hard. How do I explain our relationship during those eight years of misery? For the most part, I kind of shut Todd out. I didn't look to him for much of anything except help with Lexi so I could go to doctor's appointments and have this surgery or that surgery. I didn't confide in him. We didn't talk about things. I talked to my friends, my mom and my therapist. But not really to Todd, and he didn't talk to me either. Todd isn't known for his emotional bandwidth. He's not a touchy-feely kind of guy and doesn't want to talk about his feelings. He is a feeling stuffer and an action taker. And for the most part, that works for us. I could always count on him to be there for me and for Lexi in physical sense. He was loyal, hardworking and committed to standing by me...but in a lot of ways that wasn't all I needed. I wanted more, needed more, but he couldn't give it to me. He just wasn't capable. It just isn't him. So, I pushed him away and he pushed me away back. And by the time September 2018 rolled around, I was done with it.

We were supposed to go away to Crested Butte for the weekend on our bi-annual trip mountain biking together without Lexi. This trip always gave us a chance to connect and just be together, and we have always cherished it. But this time as I was getting ready to leave, I thought, I don't want to go. And in fact, I don't want to go anywhere with this man, not now, not ever. It hit me like a ton of bricks, like a smack in the face. I had been so wrapped up in my own life that I didn't even acknowledge how messed up our relationship had become. But here we were ready to leave, and I was feeling pretty sure we wouldn't be going to Crested Butte ever again.

I spent the entire spring and summer running away from these festering feelings. I had fallen out of love with my husband. And I resented him on so many levels. I hated him for being negative, I hated that he always worked late, I hated him for drinking too much and generally not caring about anything. But what I didn't realize at the time is even though he was quite often an asshole, I had driven him there by not recognizing his role in my recovery. I had hurt him too. I had hurt him by having a party with my girlfriends to celebrate my first year without surgery. I hurt him by telling him I didn't care if he came to Telluride to support me or not. In effect I was saying I don't need you, you don't matter. I hurt him over and over and he was unable to communicate that to me. I thought he just didn't care. We hurt each other unknowingly, indirectly, painfully. And now it was time to face it.

Todd and I have always had this rule, never go to bed mad. And we have been true to that. Even though we had our problems, no one has ever slept on the couch. It wasn't like we were fighting. We just weren't anything, we were indifferent. And I will take a good fight over indifferent any day of the week. Indifference means compliance. It means I just don't care either way. It isn't worth my time to fight with you because I don't really care about the outcome. That was where we were. Two people sharing a house, a daughter, a life without a care about our relationship. It was very, very sad.

I remember sitting on a park bench in Louisville talking to Heidi on the phone and saying, "I don't know if we can fix this." I was crying. I was hurt. My gut throbbed with the heartbeat of nausea churning in my stomach. I was devastated. I had no idea what to do. And when I went home to confront Todd, he begged me to go with him on the trip. He said we could talk, that he would change, try harder, be better. But I didn't believe him. I wanted to, but I didn't. I thought he was wired just one way and incapable of evolving. It wasn't until he spoke up after I spent hours talking about how *I felt*...It wasn't until he said, "Erin, what about me? What about how all of your suffering affected me? Don't you ever think about how hard it was on me?" Then I finally realized what was happening.

That statement eventually changed everything.

The answer to that question was not necessarily, no. But it was not an unequivocal yes, either. I mean I thought about Todd, but he always seemed so steady and even-keeled. His job was great. His bike riding talent had exploded through the roof. He seemed just fine to me. I was the one who had it hard, not him. I was the one who suffered day in and day out. I was the miserable one. I was the fighter. I won the battle. Me, me, me.

What a farce, what a sham! To think that I was the only one hurting, that I was the only warrior. Ha! So selfish. That's when I started to turn inward and check myself. Where would I be without that man, that silent supporter, that ever-present, steady calm? The answer was, I had no idea. Todd had done everything I asked him to. He had been there every step of the way. He was there when I woke up in pain and when I went to bed in pain. He was there when I was just a shell of myself. When I barely resembled the woman he married. He didn't leave me. He was the rock and I didn't even know it. Didn't give him any credit for it.

Now don't get me wrong here, Todd had been a miserable person during much of our struggle as well. But the point here is that it takes two people to fight, it takes two people to love, it takes two people to be indifferent. It always takes two.

Whenever my daughter has a problem with another kid, the first thing I ask her is, what is your role in the disagreement? What part of this is on you? And there is always something. That isn't just true for kids, or married couples, it's true for everyone.

It's hard to reflect on our own shortcomings. It is hard to believe when someone has wronged us that we might have a role in the why. It's hard to step into someone else's shoes and try to understand exactly why they feel the way they do. It takes practice. And for me, this experience with Todd opened me up to the human experience in a whole host of ways. I became a better human. I am able to take a step back and see things through a different lens. I am so much better at NOT passing judgment. I take my time before I make conclusions. I think, how did this person get here? What experience did they have that brought them to this moment? And how do I fit into that? How can I support them? How can I be there? How can I do better to understand?

Todd and I did go to Crested Butte a day late. And the repair of our marriage was not overnight. It took months of conversation and work. In a way we had to relearn how to be together without misery, drama and hardship. My health had more or less taken eight years of our ten-year marriage and thrown it in the toilet. But we did survive, and we are stronger for it.

Todd has learned to give me the verbal support I need. He tells me now that he is proud of me and my fight. He tells me that I could have a Red Bull story too! And even if that's not true, it's what I want to hear. I want him to say that I am his favorite female athlete. That he would pick me over all the rest even after everything.

He has also worked on being a better listener instead of just trying to fix everything. Sometimes now he tries so hard to listen I have to ask, "Are you listening to me? You're not saying anything." He has agreed to forgo crazy biking adventures every six months so we can have different experiences which are the ones I now crave. Since the Telluride 100 I have not raced my bike again and it has been almost two years. I wanted to show the world and myself that a miraculous comeback was possible, and I did. I got what I wanted from my bike. I was angry and the anger fueled me. I wanted to show all the haters, the people who didn't believe me; I wanted to show them I could not be beat down, that they were wrong and I was right. I did that. And after that was over, I wanted to spend vacations going to new places and seeing new things. I wanted to eat new foods, go to museums, get dressed up, and Todd was like "Wait, what?"

See he hasn't changed since the day I met him. If anything, he has become more focused on the few things that drive him—the bike, work and our family. That's it. He is pretty simple. And he likes to go to the same places and do the same things over and over. That used to be okay with me, but now I want more. I don't want to go to Crested Butte for the 500th time. I want to ride new trails, see new mountains, explore. So, we have had to compromise more. My perspective on pretty much everything has changed since I healed from all this trauma. I learned that life is completely unpredictable and even though we all "know" that, I think you have to truly live in its unpredictability to appreciate this fact. So, after this trip to Crested Butte, our next weekend getaway as a couple was in Santa Fe, New

Mexico. A place we had both never been, even though it's a short seven-hour drive from our house. We brought bikes and rode them, but we also went to the famed Meow Wolf, shopped in the downtown square, looked at crazy expensive artwork on Canyon and went out to fun, fabulous restaurants. It was great, and in the end, made us both really happy.

When we got married back in 2005 we both wrote our own vows and unveiled them on the day of the wedding. We had not shared them with one another until that fateful day. And in them, we both wrote about compromise. Both knowing how strong the other's personality was, this would be vital to our long-term success as a married couple. It was true that day and it's true now. We had no idea what we would have to face as Team Johnson, but we knew compromise would be a big part of it.

Now 3.5 years after my last surgery things are good. Our marriage is solid. The foundation like concrete. We both know that we weathered something not many people could. And that is quite satisfying. Our daughter is thriving and we are happy. We still fight, disagree and have issues, but we know our issues now are not big ones. We mostly argue about how to spend our money. For example, last year he wanted to invest in our house and I wanted to go to New Zealand. I could care less about having wood floors or new baseboards—I wanted to DO things, create memories, have experiences. However, I can be practical. And I did feel a sense of guilt for what I put Todd through. So, we did go through with a mini-remodel and it's quite lovely. Again, compromise. This year it's different. I get to choose how we spend the big bucks. I have decided on a new back deck. With the COVID-19 Pandemic in full swing, outdoor space has become very important to everyone. It's a safer place for my parents and friends to spend time with us. At first glance that might seems like a win for Todd (practical property investment), but I swear he really did leave it up to me.

Todd:

I am not sure where to start since most of this period was greyed out and the years were blurred. Every surgery ran together as did the highs and lows. It was a continual reset... surgery/ challenge > discovery to identify the new challenge > build-back > normalcy > and then challenge again.

The challenge ultimately became our normalcy. Every doctor visit, every prescription refill, every game-ready (ice machine), every mood-swing (situationally/ drug side effects), and enduring each day to get to the next. I became numb to each step of the process... doctors' visits, filling up the ice machine, insurance bills, the effects of painkillers (mental), Erin crying, and the unknown. At this point Erin was relying on the drugs to get her through the day and her mom/ friends to support her emotionally.

During this time, Lexi was our main priority and we did everything to shield her from the challenges. Secondarily for me it was work. For Erin it was her recovery (which was her central priority in many cases) understandably so... During this period, I remained as stable as I could while our world spun out of control. I did work long hours, which is my job, but it did help distract me from the chaos. However, my main outlet (then and now) has always been the bike, which sets my balance.

I would say the hardest part of this period was the mental journey. The physical part was pretty scripted even though the doctors sucked at transparency, but eight years of figuring it out got us through that part. The mental fortitude Erin needed to get out of bed every day, put a smile on her face, and act as if it was just another day took more strength than most will ever know. Sure, painkillers helped her manage/ tolerate the pain but they also clouded her brain. As soon as she could manage her pain with Advil, she stopped taking the painkillers. This was really the crux since you become mentally dependent on them. I cannot imagine how hard this was for her. Then having to do it over and over again... Total mental F/*-...

I probably do not tell her enough how proud I am of her but it is always in my head. I struggle, at times, putting my thoughts into words. For someone to persevere over the challenges she went through time and time again is better than any Red Bull "girl power" (or boy power) story I have seen. I believe in sport and in life the mental game sets the best a step above the rest. My wife has that tenfold and is unbreakable. For that, I am so proud of what she overcame and for reinventing herself every day!

CHAPTER 29

Western and Alternative Medicine

MY MOM USED to tell me necessity is the mother of invention. So, basically, when shit hits the fan, good things happen. Predominantly because there is no other choice in the matter—it's either deal and adapt or get eaten alive by your circumstances. This was definitely true for me.

In the beginning of the journey, I looked in one place for answers, and that was Western medicine. Western medicine is essentially evidenced based, conventional medicine, driven by science and the treatment of symptoms as they relate to physical systems in the body. One of the great benefits of Western medicine is that generally it is effective quickly. For example, if you go to the emergency room after falling off your bike, you can get X-rays to find out if there is a broken bone. You can get medicine for the pain and a cast to allow time for the break to heal. You are in and out in a few hours. Western medicine generally focuses on pathology; curing a particular disease or fixing a sustained trauma. The steps follow this progression with the goal of improving the patient's quality of life:

1. diagnose
2. stop disease or trauma from expanding
3. relieve symptoms of disease or trauma
4. prevent further spread of disease or trauma
5. cure or fix

And to be frank this sounds pretty good to me. It sounds direct, clear and to the point, all things that absolutely speak to my personality in general. But what happened when I followed this format and didn't fit into the mold? When doctors couldn't fix me, couldn't control my pain, couldn't prevent further trauma? I'll tell you what, they abandoned me. There were the exceptions including my primary care doctor, Dr. Omer and Dr. MK, of course. But of the over thirty doctors I visited they were the only ones who cared enough to stand by me. This fact, my friends, is a big, big problem, not just for me, but for our entire healthcare system. If only roughly 6% of doctors are standing by their patients through challenging diagnoses or complications, do we really think that is enough? What if I didn't have the financial resources to keeping fighting and searching for answers? What if I didn't have family to help with my daughter? What would have happened to me? I could still be walking around with a cane with a potentially deadly opioid dependency. This is completely unacceptable.

If you are a patient or future patient (which we all are), take the wheel and drive. Prepare yourself before your visit to the doctor (if you can). We have such a vast array of worthwhile knowledge at our fingertips. Don't be afraid to read medical journals and investigate your situation. Find reputable sources of information and educate yourself. Knowledge is power—the more you know, the more you will understand. Don't sit idly by waiting for your fifteen-minute appointment in hopes the doctor is going to provide some magic hocus pocus that will make everything bad go away. Generally, it just doesn't work like that.

Do research on your doctor too! Read their reviews, see where they went to school and how long they have been practicing. Find who is right for YOU. And if you meet with a doctor and you don't like them, go see someone else! There are good ones out there, but the chances of getting lucky the first time around are not so high. Six percent, right?

As patients, we need to get more than one opinion, always, every time. And especially when the situation is serious. I cannot stress this enough!! One of my very close friends called me several years ago and she said her son had been diagnosed with RSS (Russel Silver Syndrome). Ultimately, this meant that her son would likely only grow to be four feet eleven inches tall. She was horrified as she thought about his future and the hardships that would befall him. His diagnosis had come from one of the leading experts in the field at Children's Hospital. When we talked about it, I encouraged her to go get more opinions. She pushed back saying, "this doctor is the foremost in the field, she knows exactly what she's talking about." I told her that doesn't matter and pointed directly to my own experience. She couldn't argue with that and indeed pursued others in the field to assess his condition. And you know what, that "premier" doctor was wrong. Her son did not have RSS. Now, I am 100% sure the original doctor on the case thought she was right and had the best intentions, but doctors are human and they make mistakes. If my friend had followed the original course of treatment, things could have become quite messy for her son. Thankfully, he eventually was diagnosed with celiac disease and is growing up happy and healthy. Opinions, opinions, opinions, get them.

And if you happen to be a doctor and you are reading this, stop the madness. Trust your patients, get inquisitive, ask questions, make time to have the hard discussions. Take a picture of your patients so you can remember their faces. Treat them as human beings and mostly treat them as if you were treating your son or daughter, mother or father. And if the insurance companies, hospitals, whatever won't allow you the time you need, demand it. Make change, for God's sake, make changes. You are the heartbeat of our nations medical system, without you we all suffer. You hold the power. You are administering care, the buck stops with you.

It was Western medicine that eventually discovered the fact that my hip cup was moving in its socket. And that was, essentially, magic for me. After eighteen months of hell I had an answer and knew the doctors could fix me. But after that surgery and after the second ankle reconstruction, I was still in a dark place. It was not until I met Shaman Melissa that the rest of me healed. It was not just my body that needed fixing, it was my spirit. They were not two separate things—my body and spirit were intertwined and could not be separated. Without both being intact, I could not feel whole. I was still broken. Western medicine alone could not provide everything I needed. I had to look elsewhere for answers and there, I discovered a whole new approach to healing.

While Western medicine works to reduce or eliminate physical symptoms in the physical body, alternative medicine, whether it be Eastern medicine or Native American medicine, looks at the relationship between the physical body as it relates to its spirit or energy. Most of us grew up with Western medicine as our guide only seeking out alternatives when Western medicine fails us. It's my hope that perhaps because my full healing was not achieved until I healed my soul, that maybe you will consider looking at a bigger picture once confronted with your own tough medical choices.

I am no expert on alternative medicine. But I do know one thing for sure, we are more than our physical bodies. Our thoughts, our emotions and our spirits are all connected to our physical health. To ignore this connectedness is to only treat some of the problem. I wish I had walked down the path of spiritual healing long before I did. But just because I had a profound experience with a Shaman, doesn't mean everyone will. I don't claim to have all of the answers. I just know that I was not fully well until I addressed a different type of broken, and not one that Western medicine could diagnose and treat.

Don't be afraid to take a step back when confronting a health problem and ask tough questions about yourself. Seek help to address not just your physical issues but your mental and emotions ones as well. We are one whole person, not devoid of one aspect of the human condition. Healing can come in many forms. And healing one aspect of self can also trickle into other notable places, bringing about real lasting change. Alternative medicine is better equipped to put the puzzle pieces together because the basis for treatment looks at all aspects of the self. That doesn't mean Western medicine doesn't have a place, it surely does. But be aware of what alternatives are out there and how they might help you face your own health challenges.

CHAPTER 30

Staying Uncomfortable

AFTER THE TELLURIDE 100 and doing the work to heal my relationship with Todd, I found myself once again looking for something new. I had finally slowed down and I honestly had no idea where I would throw my unrelenting energy next. I was tired of riding my mountain bike, but couldn't go back to my old transition from biking to running. That wasn't in the cards anymore...hum, what shall I do?

Dance again? I have thought often over the years about getting back to dance, but since moving to Colorado, that idea always seemed like a waste of the space. Meaning, here I was living in one of the most beautiful, majestic places arguably in the world, and I was going to spend time in a dance studio instead of in the outdoors? Yeah, no. There were so many things that seemed inherently wrong with that choice. In addition, I was now forty-five years old and hadn't danced a step since I was, oh, twenty-three maybe. I hemmed and hawed over the idea for a few weeks and googled dance studios in Boulder and the surrounding towns. I happened upon one called "Streetside" that specialized in hip-hop style dancing, my favorite. And to my dismay they had tons of classes for adults! There was a beginner class on Tuesday at noon. Perfect, Lexi would be in school and Todd at work, so no one would really get a chance to razz me about the decision to take a dance class which was well out of my current comfort zone.

I solicited two of my friends, Juli and Melissa, to go to the class with me. It was taught by the studio's owner, Rico. Rico is like no other person you will ever meet. He has this smile that lights up the whole world and he makes everyone who walks in his studio feel special. He's a lover and a hugger and a genuinely amazing human being. But on my first day in his class, I was like, why is this guy hugging me...and why is an incredibly talented man teaching a bunch of middle-aged women in Boulder how to dance hip-hop? See, Rico had danced with talents like Britney Spears, Janet Jackson, Usher, John Legend, Michael Jackson and Prince. Seriously, this guy is no joke.

The first class was intimidating. I was nervous and I didn't want to suck, because I still hate sucking at anything. When we started, I put myself in the back, right corner and tried to follow along with the warm up. The thing about Rico's class (which I now know) is that he does the same warm up every time. But it's kind of long and everyone seems to know it. So, my tribe and I just bumbled along trying to keep up. I didn't know what was going on, and quite honestly, I felt pretty stupid. But I was there trying and he wasn't going to get rid of me that easily.

After the warm up segment, we started to learn a short "piece" or dance for the class. This time he actually taught the choreography and everyone in the class had to learn together. I felt better then. Rico's signature style included lots of fancy footwork and I did have trouble keeping up, but once he put on the music, I felt the light inside me that had been dormant for twenty-two years explode. When I look back on that fateful first class—and I remember it so vividly—I can almost feel the reignition of a passion so deep and visceral, it completely caught me off guard. This was what I wanted to do now. DANCE! DANCE! DANCE!

Of course, my husband hadn't known me when I was a dancer and my daughter had never even heard me talk about dancing, but here I was going to hip-hop class at least twice a week. Juli and Melissa didn't fall in love with Rico and Streetside that day, but I sure did and I knew if I wanted to dance again, I would have to go it alone.

Streetside really is a dance family. When people show up at the studio it seems like everyone knows everyone and they have been coming for years. For me, this was really uncomfortable. I don't like big groups of people and I'm not good at making small talk. In fact, I hate it. So, when I came to class, I didn't say anything to anyone. I just changed my shoes, went to my little spot on the right side of the room and danced. I did this for at least six months. Talked to NO ONE. But I got better and I was having a ton of fun. I got in there, got my groove on, then got out as fast as possible. I was feeling more confident and ready to try other classes, not just Rico's. I discovered other styles of hip-hop in the studio by expanding the classes I attended. Once I signed up for a workshop and when I got there I was AT LEAST twice the age of everyone in the class. I could have been any one of their mothers. I stayed for about an hour until the teacher told us to partner up…then I was like, umm, no, that is just too weird. I'm out.

But even though I was feeling good about my dancing, it was hard to not be a part of the community at the studio. I always felt like kind of an outsider. It was like being young in middle school again when all the kids around you are talking and laughing, but they aren't doing that with you. I wasn't hurt like I would have been as a kid, but it always was hard. I would get to class as late as I could and leave as soon as it was over without so much as saying hello to anyone.

Then in August 2019, Rico suggested I audition for an adult performance troupe. I was honored that he would ask me, but I immediately thought, oh no, those days are over. I do not want to get on a stage again, no interest in that. I said thanks but no thanks, it was too much of a commitment for me. When I went home and thought about it more, I considered that maybe it would be fun to learn a piece and actually get to work on it, get better and potentially make it something really special. But still, I wasn't ready for all that. I was enjoying taking classes and that was enough.

Rico:
Erin was so guarded. She just came to class with her trucker hat

pulled down low. I couldn't even see her eyes. She kept all her in-teractions short. It was clear she didn't want to make any friends. I would try and reach out to connect with her, but she gave nothing in return. So, I tiptoed around her a bit and she didn't give me the time of day. It was kind of a challenge for me. And if I am honest she reminded me a lot of myself, all quiet and private. It wasn't until Erin wrote me a Christmas card that I learned about her depth. She told me how happy she was to be dancing again and how grateful she was for the studio. I had no idea Streetside had made such an impact on her because she wouldn't let me in.

As I tried new teachers at the studio, there was one who really caught my eye. She only taught as a substitute for Rico a few times, but I really fell in love with her style. She was young, maybe twenty-two or twenty-three, but she reminded me of me a little bit at that age. Hungry, talented and wanting to do nothing but dance. I had been that girl twenty-two years ago. Now I certainly can't do every-thing I did back then, but I can hold my own in most adult classes. About four weeks after company placements were announced, this girl, Danni, took over one of the adult troupes that was flailing. The Streetside manager emailed me asking if I was interested in joining, no try-out necessary. The group would meet on Saturdays so no week night commitment needed. I thought, why not? The universe is telling me something here. Let's just do it. So, I did.

Due to a preplanned trip to Crested Butte with Todd, I was going to miss the first rehearsal, and I was all bent-out-of-shape about it. Miss the first rehearsal! What if it was really hard, what if I couldn't catch up, what if she put me in the way back, what if she put me in the front? My head was swimming with these thoughts. I was genu-inely nervous. I was so anxious about this commitment, and it was taking up way too much of my mind space. Upon our return from the mountains I met with Danni about thirty minutes early the following Saturday to learn what I had missed. Thankfully, it wasn't the end of the world after all. She had placed me on the far-left side of the stage with a seasoned company member, Adrianne, as my partner. And thank God for her. She made me feel at ease and welcome. Our theme for the upcoming show was "school house rock" or something like that and for this adult piece we were all teachers. Adrianne and I were drama teachers. There were also gym teachers, science teachers, English teachers, etc. I think there were at least ten or twelve of us total, so it wasn't going to be just me out there on stage. And for that I was incredibly grateful.

The show was scheduled for early November and because we started late, it was a big push to get the piece done. We actually finished the chorography just the week before the show. So, there was really no time to make it great. But we did it and we all worked hard in the process.

The day of the show I woke up physically ill. I was so nervous, so uncomfortable. Why was I doing this to myself? I was enjoying dancing and going to class so much. Why did I sign up for this? All of my sweet, supportive friends wanted to come, but I told them, no way. I didn't want them to come because I was already a mess of nerves, and moreover, I didn't know what was going to happen. Only Todd and Lexi were coming to this performance. And let's just call the performance what it was:

A.

Dance.

Recital.

Don't get me wrong, it was a good one, very well done. And the studio does have some incredible talent. But this was a dance recital and I was in it. Oh, my Lord.

The show was held at Boulder High School Auditorium which is actually quite nice. I think it seats around 1,000 people. The stage is big and scary. And I just felt so weird. We ran through a "mark" of our piece so we knew where our placements were on stage once the music came on. After that, we ran through a full-dress rehearsal. Our piece was almost last in the show, so I had to wait FOREVER to get this run through over with. And did I mention that this dress rehearsal was being filmed? Oh geez.

When the time came we walked out on stage in costume. My starting pose was in a runner's lunge, right foot in front bent at the knee, left leg straight in the back. And when I am standing there in my pose and waiting for the music to start, I fall fucking over. Like, fall down, right on my ass. There was no other movement on stage except me falling. Yep that really did happen. Of course, the music did start and the dancing commenced, but I was so embarrassed. That fall stayed with me throughout the whole run through. When we were done, I called Todd to check in and told him what had happened. I told him I didn't know what I was doing and this was probably a mistake. And on top of everything, I still really didn't have any dance friends and mostly hung out by myself backstage. It felt kind of stupid.

But as they say in dance recital land, the show must go on.

At 6:00 p.m. people started filing into the auditorium and I peeked out to see where Lexi and Todd were sitting. I was glad they were there no matter what happened. And I was also glad I was showing my daughter that in order to grow, you have to get uncomfortable— and uncomfortable I was. Per the show order, I had to wait for just about every other group to go before we were up. The butterflies in my stomach swirled like a tornado. I just wanted to get this over with and go the hell home.

When the time finally came, we walked out on stage and I got into my starting pose. And I stayed upright until the music started. YES! And when the beat dropped, I was transformed into a performer. I was twenty-two again in front of thousands of people. I was happy and alive. I was forty-five and I didn't care if I was good or bad or average. I was doing it. For two minutes I was in the raw moment and I had forgotten all my worries, the movements of the dance embedded in my body. When it was over and we walked off the stage I hugged Adrianne saying thank you for being my dance rock. I was so relieved I didn't screw up or fall over. But most of all, I was proud I had conquered my fear. I did it and, of course, I just couldn't wait to do it again.

Rico:

I remember that fall in the dress rehearsal, I was like "oh crap," but you showed right then and there, what a fighter you are. You killed it once you started dancing, and again that night during the performance. I was like "okay then..."

The following week when I was taking the advanced adult class at the studio, the teacher, Luz, called me out. She said, "You did great at the show, amazing. Whenever you want to join my troupe, we would love to have you." Another invitation, and this one meant a lot to me. Luz's choreography was challenging and she had me in her class many times. For her to see something in me and invite me to join—without a formal audition—the most advanced of the adult companies, I was really quite humbled. Again, I said no, with the vague explanation "Wednesday nights aren't good for me." To be frank I was intimidated by the young adults in her troupe. I was certainly at least fifteen or twenty years older than any other dancer. What if I couldn't keep up? When I told her no, she was sweet and said if I changed my mind, the offer stands.

I went home and considered her offer further...more discomfort, more challenge, more practice, more commitment. Yes! This WAS what I wanted. I had spent the last ten years suffering and now I'd found this thing, dance, that was lighting me up and filling my soul with joy. I loved working hard and being uncomfortable because that was where the magic happened.

What was I waiting for?

A week later I joined.

And on top of that I also joined Rico's group. So now I had three troupes, three teachers and three pieces to perform in the next show coming up in February 2020. I was a dancing machine and loving it. And as you know by now, when I do something, I'm all in. And with dance it was no different, I was definitely all in. The way I see things is this: if you want to be good at something, you can't just do it once a week. I don't care if it's your job, your hobby, your sport, your whatever. If you want to excel, you have to practice. I wanted to get better and grow as a dancer even though I was so damn old, not to mention all patched up and put back together. But I was willing to do the work and you know what? I got better.

For the next performance I invited everyone who wanted to come! Most of my friends came and some brought their kids and husbands. My mom, Todd and Lexi came too. I was still a bundle of nerves, but this time I was more excited than anything. I loved all of the pieces I was performing. They were all VERY different, but each spoke to me and challenged me in a different way. I just couldn't wait to get out there and dance. And when it came time for the show to start I was so ready! I boogied my little heart out. The performance went well and again I was happy. After the show was over all of my people hugged me and told me how proud they were of me. And I was proud of myself too. Who would have thought that just three years ago that day I couldn't even walk and was so out of my mind on OxyContin I barely knew my name? And here I was dancing hip-hop with twenty-somethings. It was truly remarkable.

The other thing that came out of my growing commitment to the dance studio was I finally became part of the Streetside dance family. After spending a year and a half dancing at Streetside, I had finally discovered the community there. I had made friends and connections that I still have today. And as I got closer to some of them, I started to share bits of my story. How I had lost a decade of life to pain and suffering and that now, I do what I want to do. I don't care what people think of my dancing, I love it and that's all that matters. It fills me up in way that biking or running never did. It is creative and expressive, always changing and growing. Don't get me wrong, I still ride my bike, hike, camp, etc. But more than anything at this time in my life, it is dance that I crave.

Rico:

Erin is a pusher, but in a good way. She pushes everyone around her to try new things. She is a role model for women and adults. Erin does what she wants too and she is always true to herself. She doesn't care who she is dancing with as long as she is dancing. Her energy is so different now. She has many friends at the studio and is more vulnerable, open and shares her passion with everyone around her. It is beautiful.

Life Lesson #5 – Push yourself to do what you love and continue to try new things

What fills you up?
What is something you love or have loved?
What is something that you have always wanted to try?
What have you abandoned because you thought you were too old or don't have time? Well, let me tell you the time is now.

You are not too old, too broken, too tired or too busy. There are always excuses, but they don't work here. You can find the thing that fills you up and it doesn't have to be the same thing you thought it was...you can explore, expand and open yourself up to rich, new experiences. You can reinvent yourself over and over. You can get uncomfortable and you can decide to grow. You can set an example for your children, your friends, your family. Because growth is conta-gious. Once someone sees you grow, they want to grow too. It's like a chain reaction. Be someone's inspiration, be someone's hero.

What is a hero? A hero is someone who proves to be an inspiration to us. For children and young people, heroes are usually associated with fantasy and make believe. Marvel and DC comics produce "super" heroes by the dozen. Men and women who do the right thing, fighting for freedom and justice and for people who can't fight for themselves. They are legends with just the right moral compass. For kids, these stories assume the same purpose as Bible stories. They distinctly define right from wrong and generally show that if you do the good thing, the moral thing, everything will work out in the end.

Of course, as adults we know this is total bullshit. When you grow up you learn that the good guy doesn't always win and the bad guy doesn't always go down in a flame of defeat. In the real world heroes take on a new meaning. A hero can be anyone.

I have had more than one person tell me you are my hero, you are so inspiring. And there is no question, I like hearing that, but I hardly think I am worthy of that title. I'm not fighting the good fight, I don't have a perfect moral compass. I didn't fight for anyone else, I fought for myself. I pushed and prodded, scraped and crawled just to get by, to get up, to keep moving, to keep living. I am no hero. So, when I hear people use this term to describe me I think about my own heroes and what we might have in common. How is it that people who are doing amazing things can be put into the same category with little ol' me? It just doesn't seem right.

At this moment, my biggest hero is a kid named Dior. Well, Dior isn't really a kid, he is a junior college football player on the Netflix show, Last Chance U. Last Chance U is a documentary that moves from one junior college football team to another profiling the most winning programs. They all have one thing in common, young men with big dreams to play football at a Division 1 school or in the NLF. The reasons these kids haven't made it there yet are numerous. Some of them couldn't make the grades the first go-around at a big university. Others were busted for drug use or misconduct and junior college is their second chance. Regardless, the show lets you into the lives of the coaches, the school and the players. Season five profiles Laney College and there I was introduced to Dior.

Netflix is my morning ritual. I get up about an hour or so before my family. I make coffee, black as night and eat two monster cookies. I do this every single morning and it makes me so happy. During this time, I used to catch up on work, read the depressing news or stew over social media posts. Now I watch Netflix and it is so much more fun than any of those other things. When I started season five of Last Chance U, I immediately fell in love with Dior.

Dior is a young man with stunning talent at the wide receiver position. (If you don't know anything about football, more or less this is the guy who catches the ball when the quarterback throws it). Problem is Dior is five feet eight inches tall. No coach in his (or her) right mind is going to draft a five-foot eight-inch receiver, it just ain't gonna happen. Wide receivers average six foot one, since they need to be able to jump higher than the defensive players that are trying to knock the ball out of their hands. So, the chances of Dior ever making it to the NFL are pretty slim just because he wasn't born the "right" size.

But to him, none of that matters. He has a chance to play for the state champion Laney College football program and he's going to make the most of it. In order to do that, this is what his life looks like—wake up, go to school and then to practice. After practice he goes to work from 6:00 p.m. until midnight at a fast-food restaurant called Wing-Stop. Then because he finishes so late, he doesn't want to drive back to school, so he sleeps in his car. The next day, he does it again and again and again. And he doesn't complain. You can tell he's tired, but he is also grateful. Probably grateful to be on TV, but also grateful to play and showcase his talent. And he is a beast on the field. I love him. I love everything about him.

After Laney loses the first two games of the season, they also lose their three quarterbacks to injury—THREE! That is bad luck to the nth degree. And two games into the season, the coach can't really go find another person to play this key position. So, guess who plays quarterback in game three? Yup, Dior. And he plays lights out. Now you can tell when watching the game that Laney's opponent isn't great, but that doesn't matter. This five-foot eight-inch guy who works a full-time job, goes to school, plays wide receiver and sleeps in his car is the glue that brings the team together for their first victory. And I cry big, blubbery tears on my couch at 7:00 a.m. I can't believe he pulled it off. I am so proud, I feel like his mom.

He is a hero.

How can I share that title with him? I haven't had to face even half of his hardships in my forty-seven years of life. Not even close. And then I think more deeply about why I feel like he deserves the title of hero. Number one, his attitude. He is positive and grateful. Number two, he seizes opportunity. Instead of complaining when the coach asks him to play quarterback, instead of whining about lost playing time at his regular position, he grabs the chance by the proverbial balls and takes it. Number three, he is forging his own destiny and not letting his circumstances or challenges get in the way of fighting for what he wants. And that is when is dawns on me. Everything I love about him, I also love about me, my husband, my family and my doctors.

I wasn't always this person. Well, maybe deep down I was, but it took falling on hard times to really dig deep inside myself to bring out the qualities I so love in Dior. Even now, after my nightmare has ended, I like to say I am a work in progress, always growing and changing; never satisfied and always looking for the next amazing life experience.

I have no idea what will happen to Dior throughout the rest of the season on "Last Chance U," but I hope someone, somewhere sees what I see in this young man and gives him the chance he so deserves. Dior, today you are my hero.

Epilogue

It's August 2020 and I'm packing for two solo nights in the mountains.

As I prepare for my journey, while rooting through the storage closet in our basement for camping supplies it dawns on me how many "orthopedic" aids we have down there—crutches, a walker, a wheelchair, a shower seat, shower covers for ankles, two walking boots, a "game ready" ice machine and a raised toilet seat (that one is the worst). I want to tell my friends don't go buy anything for your family members if they ever get hurt, just come to the Johnsons, we have it all! I know we have to keep it, because my time in good health is limited. Eventually, I will need more hip replacements. But man, I hate all of this stuff.

I am leaving because I've had it with life for the moment and want to check out! Covid-19 has changed everything for the world and the polarizing nature of politics and the upcoming election is exhausting. Lexi is comfortable with online school and can pretty much take care of herself. I am ready for some me time, alone amongst the deciduous forest and high peaks of Colorado. Last week as life challenges seemed to crescendo, I asked Todd if I could leave. He could tell I needed a break and granted me two nights to breathe fresh air, sleep under the stars and just be. Sometimes it's hard to know what we need to take care of ourselves, and even when we do know, sometimes it's hard to ask for it.

As I get older I am better at asking... Because I know how I come out the other side of self-care time. Whether it's a warm bath, take-out, dancing or a two-day getaway, I know that when I do these things, I am better because of it. The world is not going to stop because I do something for myself. It's not selfish to do things that make you happy. And things that make you happy don't have to involve your family, your work or your friends. They can just be for you.

And you know what happens when we take care of ourselves? We are better mothers and fathers, better daughters and sons, better employees and employers. We are better because we stopped trying to take care of everyone and everything and started to take of ourselves. When I get back from this camping trip, the silence and stillness will have revitalized me, and I will be ready to face my life and responsibilities with a renewed sense of purpose and grace. Todd has realized that this benefits him as well—when I'm in a good place it's good for our whole family.

See, Covid-19 has just pissed me off. When everything shut down in March, 2020 I was so mad. I could see that life was going to change for a very long time and I was angry. It's not fair, I told myself. I was just starting to feel good, feel great! I was dancing and riding my bike. I was strong and happy. I cried heaving sobs in the bathroom, mourning another setback to living life to my fullest potential. I had already lost a fucking decade…and now I had to lose more. *It's not fair. It's not fair. It's not fair.* I wasn't buying into "we are all in this together." Where was the whole world when I spent ten years suffering? I will tell you where it was, just moving right along. The world forgot about me. The world had hiking groups, activities and vacations while I had pain, pills and surgeries. I wanted my life to be normal. I had already been quarantined and miserable. I was so, so unhappy. And then came the guilt.

Guilt is a funny thing. Guilt results from doing or feeling something, reflecting upon it, then feeling bad that you thought or did that thing. What a waste of time! What's done is done. Feeling guilty about it isn't going to change it, it's just going to make you feel bad. Instead I always try to just move forward in a more authentic way, course correcting for my less desirable thoughts or actions. Always forward, never backward. But with Covid, I couldn't shake the guilt. My husband and I both kept our jobs during the shutdown and ultimately both of our industries are thriving as more people are riding bikes and getting outside. Plus, we live in a Bernie Sanders state, meaning there is a lot of social consciousness here. People feel responsible for one another and try hard to curb the spread of the disease. Our community has been quite successful up to this point in doing so.

This is not true for the rest of the country. Millions of people have lost their jobs and livelihoods, and over 200,000 people had died in the United States at this point. That's 200,000 mothers, fathers, children, friends, co-workers, souls. It's a horrible time for humanity and I am thinking about that fact that I can't dance in a dance recital. Damn. It really doesn't get more pathetic than that. And that is when the guilt creeps in. But then it dawns on me…

Life Lesson #6 – It's okay to feel what I feel

It's okay to be sad and mourn the loss of normalcy. It's okay to be mad. It doesn't mean I don't feel something for all of those suffering more in this crisis than I am. It just means that my experiences are uniquely my own. I don't need to feel guilty. I get to feel everything just the way I do. We all get this opportunity to sit with our emotions and let them just be what they are. Then we also have the opportunity to move through them and move forward.

Now, I no longer feel angry or mad. I feel patient and grateful. Life has had to slow way down and Covid has challenged our family to prioritize the most important things in our lives. We have decided where we take "risks" and where we do not. We have had to decide what feels comfortable for our immediate family, while considering the repercussions for my parents and our friends who are immune compromised. We have to consider our actions as they ripple out into the world, and that has been the biggest wake-up call.

I have always believed in fate, if you will, a universal plan for me that is mine to walk and experience. But that plan can only be put into motion through and with the actions of all other pieces of the universe moving together. Covid exposes this in the most vivid way. We are all intrinsically connected to each other. We are all walking alone, but also walking together through our lifetime. I am grateful to be part of this connected planet and even though I am sometimes disappointed with its direction, I am still happy to be here.

A little over three years ago I thought I might want to die rather than continue to live in pain. That feels like an eternity ago. Today as I sit here at a picnic table tucked away in the Colorado mountains I am in awe of the vastness of the earth and my teeny-tiny presence on it. Sometimes my feelings are so big and overwhelming, I believe they might swallow me whole. But when I am out here my perspective shifts and I am at peace.

This upcoming November I am going to be forty-eight years young. When I think about those forty-eight years, I see a life worth living. I have zero regrets. Moving forward, I do not plan to take my foot off the gas pedal. I plan to continue to live life to the fullest, to challenge myself, to grow, to change, to try new things, to evolve. My decade of crisis has made me the person I am today and I like myself so much better than ever.

I appreciate.
I accept.
I am grateful.
I am vulnerable.
I am me.
I wouldn't change a thing.

CPSIA information can be obtained
at www.ICGtesting.com
Printed in the USA
LVHW110326040821
694386LV00004B/97

9 781977 244154